The
Immunization
Decision

The Immunization Decision

A Guide for Parents

Randall Neustaedter

THE FAMILY HEALTH SERIES
North Atlantic Books
Homeopathic Educational Services
Berkeley, California

The Immunization Decision: A Guide for Parents

ISBN 1–55643–071–X

Publishers' addresses:

North Atlantic Books
2800 Woolsey Street
Berkeley, California 94705

Homeopathic Educational Services
2124 Kittredge Street
Berkeley, California 94704

Cover photograph by Carol Knight, M.D.
Cover and book design by Paula Morrison
Typeset by Campaigne and Associates

The Immunization Decision: A Guide for Parents is sponsored by the Society for the Study of Native Arts and Sciences, a nonprofit educational corporation whose goals are to develop an ecological and crosscultural perspective linking various scientific, social, and artistic fields; to nurture a holistic view of arts, sciences, humanities, and healing; and to publish and distribute literature on the relationship of mind, body, and nature.

Library of Congress Cataloging-in-Publication Data
Neustaedter, Randall.
    The immunization decision: a guide for parents/Randall
Neustaedter.
        p.   cm.
    Includes bibliographical references (p.   ).
    ISBN 1-55643-071-X : $8.95
    1. Immunization of children—Popular works.   I. Title.
RJ240.N47   1990
614.4'7—dc20   90-7029
                                                              CIP

Dedicated to my wife Susan
and my children, Fena, Althea, and Aaron,
who have made the immunization decision
a personal one for me.

Contents

Preface

The immunization decision faces every parent very soon after a child's birth. Most parents are ill-equipped to make this decision and must accept the counsel of their child's health care provider. The current massive effort to vaccinate all children in the United States usually results in a predetermined decision, yet at the same time, there is growing concern among health professionals and the public about the safety of routine immunization. Unfortunately, information about the vaccines is not generally available.

Parents have the responsibility to provide the best health care possible for their child. They must decide whether it is better for their child's health to give the vaccines or not. If parents question the validity or wisdom of administering vaccines to their child, they receive little support in their efforts to make an informed decision. This book is intended to help parents who do question the wholesale policy of mass immunization and its effect on their child.

This book has two functions. One is to give information about the diseases, the vaccines, and their side effects. The potential side effects of vaccines usually are hidden from parents. Medical professionals have often stated that broadcasting side effects of vaccines to the public would cause unnecessary concern among parents and hinder the vaccine campaign. Dr. Paul Meier summarized this position quite clearly in a panel

discussion on the efficacy of the polio vaccine campaign of
the 1950s:

> It is hard to convince the public that something is good.
> Consequently, the best way to push forward a new program
> is to decide on what you think the best decision is and not
> question it thereafter, and further, not to raise questions
> before the public or expose the public to open discussion
> of the issues (Intensive Immunization Programs, Hearings,
> 1962).

The recent passage by Congress of the National Vaccine
Injury Compensation Act has required more disclosure about
vaccines and encouraged informed consent, but parents still
have little information about the vaccines, and suppression of
information remains a goal of many pharmacies and pediatrician organizations. For example, when the American Academy
of Pediatrics' former president, Dr. Martin Smith, reviewed
information brochures for parents prepared by the U.S. Department of Health and Human Services, he recommended that
they be simplified. He said, "The length and complexity of
the materials . . . would confuse many parents and could even
needlessly alarm them" (AAP News, 1989). Parents are hungry
for information about the vaccines, especially their side
effects. They are unwilling to blindly accept the opinions of
doctors concerning medical care. This book seeks to provide
information which is usually unavailable to parents.

The second goal of the book is to give support to those
parents who choose not to immunize according to the recommended schedule. There are many good reasons why a parent
may choose to delay immunization or refuse specific vaccines.
This should be an informed decision and not one made impul-
sively or rebelliously. They need to know the side effects of
vaccines, and this information is emphasized in this book. I
present the ideas and facts here as I usually do with parents
in my office. I give the facts about diseases and vaccines,
include a summary of information about each disease, and

give parents options regarding individual vaccines as well as my recommendations. Each parent must decide what is best for each child. The text is addressed to parents. It will, I hope, serve as guide and support in the difficult immunization decision.

I recommend that parents read at least the Introduction and Conclusion of this book to understand the issues involved in making their decision. Then the pertinent chapters can be read or skimmed as the need arises to make a decision about each individual vaccine.

Previous editions of this text were published as a booklet-titled "Immunizations: Are They Necessary?" I wish to thank the practitioners at the Hering and Hahnemann homeopathic clinics for their support, editorial suggestions, and revisions of that pamphlet. In particular, Nancy Herrick, Stephen Cummings, Dana Ullman, Andrea Laurence, Dr. Harris Coulter, and Dr. Kenneth Stoller have contributed significantly through their review of the manuscript. All of the parents in my practice have been instrumental in clarifying my thinking about vaccines. Their questions have urged me on and inspired the writing of this book.

PART I:

The Decision

Introduction: How to Decide

The subjective experience of childhood vaccination is not pleasant. Babies scream and develop fevers with the first illness of their lives. Preschoolers learn fear of the doctor because they are stabbed with needles whenever they go for well-child check-ups. Older children, at least the oppositional ones, often run around the doctor's office refusing to be poked. Others refuse to talk and cling to their mothers in abject terror awaiting the dreaded needle. Parents must tolerate all of this for the good of their child. In addition, they are informed that vaccines may permanently damage their child's nervous system. This causes understandable apprehension in everyone. Parents are convinced that all of this is worth it. Or are they? Most have doubts, but little information. They have been told that vaccines are the greatest achievement of modern preventive medicine. The polio epidemic of the 1950s, the March of Dimes, and the eradication of smallpox are historical events of the recent past. We are assured that one more generation of vaccines will eliminate whooping cough, measles, and mumps as threats to our children, just as polio and diphtheria have disappeared into memory. This is a reassuring and convincing argument. Risk a few cases of rare side effects to eliminate these serious and life-threatening diseases. But lingering doubts remain.

Parents must accommodate themselves to the vaccines' side effects. They must steel themselves against their children's inevitable anxiety about the doctor visit and dread of the shot. They wonder about the publicized cases of vaccine-damaged children. Measles and mumps were simple childhood diseases once. Why all the excitement about them now? Parents are upset when their child develops a fever after a shot, though it usually is not serious. Parents are devastated if their child develops polio, seizures, or retardation after a vaccine, but these reactions are relatively uncommon. We are told that this is the price we pay for eliminating these diseases from our population. We are reassured that the incidence of these problems would be higher from the natural diseases if the vaccines were not given routinely. What is the truth about the vaccine campaign? Isn't someone making a lot of money from these millions of shots? Most parents put these doubts aside and rationalize: My pediatrician would not be influenced by a drug company's desire for profit. He would not recommend these vaccines unless he were convinced that they are necessary. I have to leave the decision to him. I just don't know enough to make a judgment about such an important issue.

As a parent you are faced with many decisions soon after your baby is born. Most of these are retractable. You can decide to use cloth diapers after four months of plastic ones. If you say the wrong thing to your child, you can recant. If you decide that giving ice cream to Jennifer for breakfast so she gets at least a little protein is not such a great idea after all, you can change your mind tomorrow. Even medical decisions are usually reversible. The decongestant makes Jesse too groggy; let's try a vaporizer tonight. But some medical decisions are momentous. Should we circumcise, should we immunize? These are weighty issues with permanent effects.

You must rely on various advisors to give you their opinions. Family, friends, and health professionals can all be helpful and informative. But you can take responsibility for the ultimate decisions. The factors that comprise medical decisions are not out of your reach. Except for emergency situations which require immediate action, you can discover the issues and weigh the pros and cons of a medical decision. Some of these may be obvious and simple, others may be agonizing. Any decision will be easier if you have support and reassurance that you are doing the right thing. Unfortunately, the subject of immunization often involves heated emotions and recriminations.

I encourage parents to gather information from professionals with differing views about immunizations. The medical issues are controversial, and you need to be aware of these controversies when making a truly informed decision about your child's health care. Individuals with differing perspectives will examine the same data and arrive at different conclusions. For that reason I have included here reviews of the medical literature for parents to examine themselves. I also recommend that parents read the chapter on immunizations in Dr. Robert Mendelsohn's book, *How to Raise a Healthy Child . . . In Spite of Your Doctor*. In addition, *Mothering* magazine and the newsletter "The Doctor's People" both publish a set of reprints on immunizations (see Resources). These publications are all generally critical of immunizations for children. Pediatricians and books on child health care are good alternative sources for pro-vaccination information.

I recommend that parents take a careful look at the vaccine question in general and each vaccine individually before making a decision for their child. In the following sections of this book I outline a practical approach that should help guide you through the maze of the vaccine question.

Three steps are necessary for parents who want to make an informed decision.

1) Get information about the vaccines.
2) Decide which vaccines you do or don't want.
3) If you decide to vaccinate, then choose the right time.

It comes as a surprise to some parents that they can choose to have one or some immunizations and refuse others. It may be difficult to find a medical provider who is willing to accept the parents' decision to give only one vaccine and not others, but finding that practitioner should prove rewarding in many ways. The side effects of some vaccines are more dangerous than others. Some of the diseases themselves are dangerous and others are benign. Each vaccine should be chosen or rejected based on your individual needs.

It is not necessary to begin giving vaccines at two months of age. Delaying immunizations will give you time to make your decision. It will also give your baby's body a chance to develop a more mature immune system and nervous system, making them less susceptible to the vaccines' toxic effects. Delay of DTP immunization until two years of age in Japan has resulted in a dramatic decrease in vaccine side effects. During the period 1970 through 1974, when DTP vaccine was begun at 3 to 5 months of age, the Japanese national compensation system paid claims for 57 permanent severe vaccine reactions and 37 deaths. During the following six-year period, 1975 through 1980, when DTP vaccine was begun at 24 months of age, severe reactions were reduced to a total of eight with three deaths (Noble *et al.*, 1987). This is an 85 to 90 percent reduction in severe reactions and deaths calculated according to total doses of vaccine administered during these years. Dr. James Cherry and colleagues reporting the American Academy of Pediatrics Task Force on Pertussis findings conclude, "It is clear that delaying the initial vaccination until a child is 24 months . . . reduces most of the temporally associated severe adverse events" (Cherry *et al.*, 1988).

Only one of the diseases for which vaccines are available commonly causes significant problems within the first year of life—whooping cough (pertussis). If you decide not to give that vaccine because of its associated dangers, then there is no harm in delaying other immunizations until your child is beyond infancy and less vulnerable to side effects of the shots.

Exposure to tetanus is extremely unlikely until your child is 2 years old, when he or she encounters situations where cuts and scrapes occur. There is no reason to begin tetanus toxoid before 2 years of age.

*   *   *

A rational and personal decision about immunizations will be possible if you follow the steps outlined in Table 1. If you consider each of these issues, then your decision will be based on facts rather than belief, propaganda, or pressure.

TABLE 1
Factors for parents to consider about immunizations

1. Individual disease incidence and severity
2. Vaccine side effects
3. Access to homeopathic medical care

---

(1) Individual disease incidence and severity

Each disease should be considered one by one. A discussion of the incidence of each disease is included in the sections which follow. Smallpox vaccination was stopped in the United States when the disease disappeared and the number of serious vaccine reactions outweighed any benefit from the immunization. We may have a similar situation with other vaccines. For example, the incidence of diphtheria and polio have declined to near zero in the United States.

The severity of the diseases must also be considered. Risking a serious vaccine reaction in order to prevent a mild childhood disease may not be the best alternative for your child. On the other hand, preventing a potentially life-threatening disease may be worth the risk of the vaccine if your child has a significant chance of exposure. For example, a child who lives on a farm or works with horses has more risk of tetanus exposure than a child in an urban or suburban environment. Travel to a foreign country may involve exposure to new diseases that a child has never before encountered. The likelihood of exposure should then be investigated and vaccines reconsidered as part of the trip plans.

(2) Vaccine side effects

Many of the vaccines have significant side effects. These can be separated into two groups: (a) immediate reactions, and (b) delayed reactions and permanent disabilities. Immediate reactions include fevers, allergic reactions and convulsions. With some vaccines, these can be quite severe. Delayed and permanent reactions include epilepsy, mental retardation, learning disabilities, and paralysis. The risks from the diseases should be weighed against the risk of these vaccine side effects. They are reviewed in the sections on individual vaccines. In addition, there are theories that immunizations are capable of initiating subtle and long-term damaging effects on the immune system and nervous system. These warrant some discussion here.

Critics of immunizations have asserted that vaccines are capable of causing recurrent respiratory infections in children because they weaken the immune system. Dr. Richard Moskowitz, noted homeopathic physician and outspoken critic of vaccines, has proposed a possible mechanism for this effect. He suggests that the vaccine may be incorporated into the body's own cells where it is capable of continually stimulating antibody production. Various kinds of naturally occurring viruses are stored within the cells of certain individuals and are associated with chronic diseases (herpes, tumors, panencephalitis). Vaccines could conceivably cause similar phenomena if they are stored within the cells. The constant sensitization of the immune system to the vaccine components within the body's own cells may weaken our natural ability to fight off other viruses and may cause an autoimmune response which could lead to serious problems.

The latent virus survives as a clearly "foreign" element with the cell, which means that the immune system must continue to try to make antibodies against it, insofar as it can still respond to it at all. Because the virus is now permanently incorporated within the genetic material of the cell, these antibodies will now have to be directed against the cell itself.

The persistence of live viruses or other foreign antigens within the cells of the host therefore cannot fail to provoke *auto-immune* phenomena, because destroying the infected cells is now the only possible way that this constant antigenic challenge can be removed from the body. Since routine vaccination introduces live viruses and other highly antigenic material into the blood of virtually every living person, it is difficult to escape the conclusion that a significant harvest of auto-immune diseases must automatically result (Moskowitz, 1983; see Resources).

Our understanding of these processes is very limited, and the long-term effects of persistent circulating antigen in the body are unknown. It may cause a continual immune suppression, which disables the body's ability to react normally to disease. Many critics have suggested taking a much more cautious approach to immunizations until we know more about possible long-lasting detrimental effects.

The possible long-term neurologic effects of the vaccines have been well documented by Dr. Harris Coulter in his book *The Assault on the American Child: Vaccination, Sociopathy, and Criminality*. He delineates a hydra-headed syndrome of brain insult and injury possibly caused by vaccines. These effects include allergies, autism, dyslexia, learning disabilities, behavior disorders, and antisocial syndromes, all attributable to the assault of vaccines on the body. He postulates that vaccines have a damaging effect on the developing myelination process of the nervous system in children. This assault causes an allergic encephalitis (inflammation or infection of the brain) with widespread effects. That is, the allergic response initiated by a vaccine injected into the body is capable of causing encephalitis and brain damage, because the physical development of nerves is disrupted. Coulter suggests that the developmental problems caused by vaccines occur in a large (and unknown) percentage of children. He speculates that the 50 percent of children who experience fever (accompanied by fussiness or screaming) after a DTP shot actually have a subtle form of encephalitis and subsequent minimal brain damage. He points out the tragic irony of giving a dangerous vaccine to prevent disease-associated encephalitis, and achieving the result of an insidious and permanent vaccine-associated encephalitis syndrome. His theories are based on the coincidence of the dramatic increase in the conditions he reports—autism, minimal brain damage, and learning disorders—since the introduction of vaccines. Coulter unequivocally blames childhood vaccines for the "new morbidity" of learning disabilities and behavioral disturbances.

> The physician is irresistibly impelled to characterize the "new morbidity" as "emotional" because these disabilities can then be blamed on the child or the parents. In fact, the responsibility should be placed squarely at the physician's own door. The vaccination program is intrinsically dangerous, which was never recognized or admitted . . . (Coulter, 1990).

Coulter points out that no studies have been conducted to investigate the association of learning disorders and other modern brain dysfunctions with vaccines. The dramatic and immediate damaging effects of vaccines are denied by vaccine proponents. It is little wonder that wholehearted disinterest is generated by the possibility of long-term nervous system sequelae. Nonetheless, Coulter's arguments for a direct association between vaccines, encephalitis, allergies, and neurodevelopmental delays are compelling.

(3) Homeopathic Medical Care

Homeopathy is a system of natural medicine that has become highly developed and accepted in England, France, Germany, South America, and Russia. In the United States, homeopathic medical care is less generally available, though it was quite prevalent and popular during the nineteenth century. Practitioners of homeopathic medicine assert that homeopathy provides effective treatment for most common childhood diseases. Homeopaths treated measles, mumps, and whooping cough during the 1800s, long before vaccines or antibiotics were available. Clinical studies have not been conducted to document the success of homeopathic treatment in these diseases or in the prevention of disease complications. Nonetheless, practitioners of homeopathy claim success and express confidence in their treatments based on 200 years of clinical experience.

Conventional medicine has little to offer when viral diseases occur, and non-homeopathic physicians are anxious to prevent what they cannot treat. The urge to immunize children is much stronger when adequate treatment is not readily available. Homeopathic medical providers express confidence in their ability to treat viral diseases and prevent complications of most childhood illnesses. They tend to have less anxiety than conventional physicians about disease complications. If the diseases are less threatening under their care, then the impetus to vaccinate children will be less compelling, especially when the potential for serious side effects exists in the vaccines.

Historically, homeopathic treatment has proved effective in a wide range of acute illnesses. During the nineteenth century, homeopathy gained general acceptance because of its ability to cure infectious diseases. During the yellow fever epidemic of the late nineteenth century in the United States, homeopathy was exceptionally effective compared to the conventional treatment of the time. A report of the Homeopathic

Yellow Fever Commission showed that in New Orleans homeopathic treatment resulted in a mortality of 5.6 percent of cases
and 7.7 percent of cases in the rest of the South. This compared
to an overall death rate of at least 16 percent (American Institute of Homeopathy, 1880). A comparison of mortality rates
among homeopathic and conventional medical treatment in the
United States and Europe in 1900 showed a two to eightfold
reduction in deaths from life-threatening infectious diseases
among the homeopathically treated cases (Bradford, 1900).
During the severe influenza epidemic of 1918, homeopathic
treatment also resulted in a significant reduction in mortality.
These results led to a wide acceptance of homeopathic treatment among the public. Although these studies were conducted in the nineteenth century, prior to the era of double
blind, controlled clinical trials, they serve as a landmark for
the recognition of homeopathy as a medical science.

Clinical studies are once again showing the effectiveness
of homeopathy—now in carefully controlled trials. Recent
publications in the *British Medical Journal*, *Lancet*, and *Nature*
are paving the way for more widespread acceptance of homeopathy and recognition of its ability to effectively treat
diseases.

Homeopathy is a medical system that uses natural substances (plant, mineral, and animal products) that purportedly
stimulate a healing reaction within the body and encourage a
curative response to illness. This theoretical framework of cure
is in distinction to that of allopathic or conventional medications which suppress the body's reactions or kill bacteria. Conventional medicines are prescribed with little regard for their
detrimental effects on the body. The benefit of the drug is
considered worth the risk of side effects. Homeopathic practitioners claim that their medications have no side effects
because they are so dilute. Homeopaths assert that the
medicines work because of their ability to trigger a reaction
within the body. The medicine is a catalyst. The healing reaction manifests as a gentle and efficient cure. This has been the

claim of homeopathy since its inception. Curative response, according to homeopaths, is not limited to the type of organism responsible for disease. It is assumed to work as well for viral as for bacterial infection. A single dose or a few doses of a homeopathic medicine are usually prescribed to trigger the desired response within the body. The minimal dose possible is employed to effect a cure.

Homeopathic medicine has several practical points which distinguish it from the methods of conventional medicine. A homeopathic medicine is chosen to treat a case of illness when it corresponds to the symptoms of the illness in the individual patient. Medicines are prescribed for the individual and not for the disease. Several different cases of ear infection or measles may require different homeopathic medicines. This is an important practical point. The symptoms of the individual, in their details and qualities, are compared to the complex of symptoms characteristic of a medicine. When the right match is made and the correct medicine is taken, the curative response begins. In a serious illness, the medicine may need to be changed as symptoms change. The services of a skilled homeopath are required in order to make these decisions.

Homeopathic theory assumes that any drug treatment will either enhance or suppress immune system function. According to homeopaths, any drug will either have a strengthening or weakening effect on the body. Since homeopathic medicines are intended to stimulate the immune system, homeopaths claim that acute illnesses resolve quickly when the body's fight against the disease is strengthened by the correct medicine. The result is a stronger immune system and resolution of the acute illness without resultant complications. In chronic conditions the body is purportedly encouraged by the appropriate homeopathic medicine to develop a higher level of resistance and less susceptibility to illness.

Homeopaths are generally concerned that antibiotics and immunizations will suppress the body's fight against disease. Dr. Richard Moskowitz has proposed that immunizations may work through a continuous suppressive process. That is, the vaccine stored within the body's cells continually suppresses the ability to respond to a viral or bacterial attack (Moskowitz, 1983).

Several cautions about homeopathic medicines are usually offered by professional practitioners. Although homeopathic medicines are available without prescription, it is advisable to seek medical care from a qualified homeopath whenever a potentially serious acute illness occurs. Various combination homeopathic medicines are also available and these are labeled with indications for symptoms such as coughs, colds, teething, etc. They are not recommended because the correct homeopathic medicine must be chosen carefully. It is unlikely that a medicine which is not prescribed appropriately for the individual case of illness will act curatively. It is possible for parents to learn to prescribe for simple acute illnesses in their child. Several books are available to help guide parents in the proper use of homeopathic treatment at home. The book *Everybody's Guide to Homeopathic Medicines* provides indications for the correct use of homeopathy in simple illnesses (see Resources). It provides guidelines for safe treatment and the appropriate times to seek professional medical care. Serious illness always requires consultation with a trained medical practitioner.

There are times when antibiotics or other medications are needed for infectious diseases, and a homeopathic or conventional medical provider can help make these treatment decisions. Tetanus is an example of a disease that requires vigorous, active treatment. It is mandatory that anyone who acquires tetanus receive conventional allopathic care and hospitalization. Similarly, any child who contracts one of the potentially serious diseases of childhood should be evaluated by a qualified medical care provider. He or she will observe your child for complications and the need for intervention.

Conventional Vaccines

Before considering each vaccine individually, some general points about vaccine effectiveness should be raised. Critics have charged that adequate studies of vaccine efficacy have not been conducted. The late Dr. Robert Mendelsohn, noted pediatrician, repeatedly questioned the use of any vaccine which has not been tested in a placebo controlled or longitudinal study of vaccinated vs unvaccinated groups. Very few studies of this kind have been conducted.

Some recent studies have shown a lack of vaccine effectiveness. For example, one researcher found a fivefold risk of *Hemophilus influenzae* b meningitis in children vaccinated against this disease compared to unvaccinated controls (Osterholm *et al.*, 1988).

Public health authorities cite the decline in disease occurrence as proof that a vaccine works. In fact, most of the diseases in question have either steadily declined since the advent of general sanitation measures during the twentieth century, or gone through waxing and waning occurrence during epidemic cycles. Critics point out that a coincidental reduction in the number of cases following vaccine introduction in a community does not necessarily prove a relationship to the vaccine. One set of statistics frequently used to document vaccine efficacy is the increase in pertussis (whooping cough) incidence when vaccine administration is stopped or decreased. This has occurred in Britain, Japan and Sweden (Cherry *et al.* 1988). Many critics, however, charge that during times of vaccine reduction, physician sensitivity to the disease increases and every lingering cough is then reported as pertussis, thereby inflating the actual number of cases (Coulter & Fisher, 1985). This possibility of heightened awareness and bias has also been considered in relation to the polio statistics during the 1950s epidemic. When the vaccine was introduced, cases previously reported as polio were now given another diagnosis, such as encephalitis. This resulted in an apparent decline in the number of polio cases (see Polio section).

Vaccine proponents assure us the vaccines are safe because side effects are rare. This statement arises from the many studies which have investigated vaccine reactions. But the validity of these studies is severely hampered by two limitations. First, most of them have examined the occurrence of symptoms immediately following the vaccine's administration. Often this period has been limited to *two days*. Some studies have extended this period to a week or two. Any delayed reaction will not be observed in such a study. In fact, delayed reactions and long-term effects are difficult to document. No studies have compared developmental or cognitive function in vaccinated and unvaccinated children.

The second important limitation of these studies involves the control group. In all of the studies, the side effects in a group of children who receive a specific vaccine are compared to the occurrence of these symptoms in a control group. The problem is that the control group is also vaccinated. If the side effect under consideration is epilepsy or developmental delays, then the control group must be unvaccinated, because any of the vaccines may be capable of inducing these problems. One cannot compare vaccinated children with other vaccinated children and hope to arrive at a valid estimate of the percentage that experience a side effect.

The problems with evaluating vaccine efficacy and safety are summarized in Table 2.

TABLE 2
Difficulties tracking vaccine efficacy and safety

1. Decline in disease occurrence prior to vaccine introduction

2. Contradictory findings of vaccine efficacy studies

3. Bias in reporting diseases when vaccines are begun or stopped in a community

4. Deficiencies of studies evaluating vaccine side effects: observation period too short and inappropriate control groups

Homeopathic Vaccines

Vaccines are available in homeopathic form, and practitioners of homeopathic medicine assert that homeopathic treatment itself also affords some protection from disease. Homeopaths suggest that children who receive ongoing homeopathic medical care are less likely to contract serious diseases and will have less complications when childhood diseases do occur. Homeopathy claims to support the immune system's functioning, and the plentiful examples of cured cases of allergy and recurrent infection in children in the homeopathic literature seem to support this contention. Since homeopathic medicines purportedly work by stimulating the body's defense mechanisms, proponents claim that serious diseases and complications of more common diseases are less likely to occur after homeopathic treatment.

Homeopathic vaccines have been prepared according to homeopathic pharmaceutical standards, and these preparations are sometimes used preventively. These vaccines have never been rigorously tested. Nonetheless, there is some evidence suggesting that homeopathic vaccines do act to prevent diseases during epidemics. One study observed the occurrence of meningitis in a group of children who received a homeopathic preventive during a 1974 epidemic in Brazil. The homeopathic group had significantly less meningitis than the unvaccinated controls (Castro & Nogueira, 1975). Other studies of whooping cough (English, 1987a), influenza (Faculty Review of Asian Influenza, 1958) and polio (Eisfelder, 1961) also suggest some protective effect from homeopathic preparations during epidemics of these diseases. For example, a study of 694 children given homeopathic *Pertussin* as a preventive for whooping cough suggested that the vaccine was at least 50 percent effective in preventing disease when incidence was compared to the general unvaccinated population (English, 1987a). This was not a controlled study. It was intended to serve as a pilot for a larger study and suggested to the investigators that such a study was warranted.

Alternative vaccines in homeopathic form are available for long-term prevention, but in the absence of any evidence of ongoing immunity from these preparations, I cannot advise their use. Several protocols exist for the administration of homeopathic immunizations for whooping cough, meningitis, diphtheria, polio, and other diseases during infancy. No long-term studies have been conducted to evaluate their efficacy, and there is no reason to suspect these vaccines continue to act preventively years after administration. In addition, disagreement exists among homeopathic practitioners about the safety and validity of introducing a homeopathic medication into the body if there are no clear indications for its use. In general, homeopathic medicines are prescribed on the basis of existing symptoms. These symptoms will guide the prescriber to the correct prescription. If a homeopathic medicine is prescribed incorrectly it could interfere with the action of other correct prescriptions or disturb the energetic balance of the organism. Classical homeopaths rely upon their treatment to develop a strong immune system. Other immune-enhancing factors in a child's life may also influence the body's response to disease and help prevent serious problems.

Legal Requirements

Legal requirements concerning immunization vary from state to state. All fifty states have compulsory vaccination laws, though the specific requirements differ. This means that parents who decide not to give the vaccines to their children will need to seek a legal exemption. All fifty states also have a medical exemption. If a physician thinks your child should not have the vaccine, then he or she can sign a waiver. Many doctors are willing to sign these, especially if they think the vaccines may have unknown long-term effects which could be detrimental to your child's health. All states except West Virginia and Mississippi have legal exemption from vaccination on the basis of parents' religious beliefs. Recent legal precedents have established that religious belief may be personal, and parents need not be associated with a religious institution opposed to vaccination. Twenty-two states have the option of personal or philosophical belief exemptions. Parents, in these cases, must sign a form or write a letter that states they are opposed to vaccines for religious or philosophical reasons. Parents need only request the immunization exemption form at their school district office when enrolling their child in school. Children cannot be refused admission to public schools if their parents have one of these legal exemptions. You can learn about your state law and exemptions by contacting the immunizations section of your State Health Department.

Private schools can set their own requirements for admission. Daycare centers, preschools, nursery schools and private elementary schools can refuse admission to any child for any reason they choose. Most of these facilities, however, are willing to abide by the recommendations of State Health Departments concerning immunization requirements. A physician's medical exemption should be an adequate waiver in all states, and in states with provisions for religious or philosophical exemptions a parent's signed statement should suffice. If the director of a private school or daycare center is hesitant about admitting your child, then he or she should be encouraged to contact the medical director of immunizations at the State Health Department. Refusal to admit a child on the basis of "inadequate" immunization could create a legal liability for a private school in a state where religious or philosophical exemptions exist. That is, parents could take a school to court if the school refuses admission to their child in a state that has these personal belief exemptions.

Many attorneys and individuals are working to ensure freedom of choice in the area of child immunization. One organization in particular, Dissatisfied Parents Together (DPT), has been instrumental in passage of legislation which protects children and their parents (see Resources). If a parent makes the choice to avoid a required vaccine, then support for that decision is available. Several court cases have provided precedents for a parent's right to make an informed decision about vaccines. The DPT organization provides a valuable service as an information center for concerned parents.

Factors that Affect the Immune System

No discussion of immunization would be complete without considering the factors that strengthen immune system functions. Several of these influences are under a parent's direct control. For example, breastfeeding protects babies from many infections. The immunoprotective value of breastmilk is unquestionable, but incompletely understood. Immunoglobulins in human milk provide passive protection from bacteria. White blood cells in human milk will actively ingest bacteria that invade the infant's body. In addition, lymphocytes carrying specific antibodies pass through breastmilk to the baby. Several other chemicals in breastmilk (lactoferrin and lysozyme) protect the breastfeeding child from infection by destroying or inhibiting growth of bacteria (Goldman *et al.*, 1982). Many other resistance factors in breastmilk (including interferon) assist the child's developing immune system function (Chandra, 1978).

A person's nutritional status is one of the prime determinants of his or her general resistance. Malnutrition and undernutrition in underdeveloped countries contribute to low resistance and a higher prevalence of infectious diseases. Similarly, the introduction of refined and processed foods will lower the resistance of a population in a developing country and cause epidemics. Good nutrition lays the groundwork for a strong immune system in your child. This includes reliance upon natural foods and avoidance of chemicals and refined products. Fresh fruits and vegetables provide essential nutrients for the growing child. Processed foods such as canned vegetables have less vitamins and altered forms of these nutrients.

Babies should be fed cooked fresh vegetables rather than prepared baby foods whenever possible. The gradual introduction of solids in the form of fresh vegetables, fruits, and grains to supplement breastfeeding (or formula if necessary) during the second six months of life will help develop immune system strength and avoid the weakening effects of food allergies. Each new food should be introduced alone to observe for allergic reactions over several days before starting another. The introduction of potentially allergenic foods too early during an infant's development may predispose him or her to allergic reactions. Avoidance of dairy products, wheat, and egg whites is advisable until a baby has been eating solid foods for at least several months. If a family history of allergies is present, then these foods should be avoided until 12 months of age. Food allergies may predispose children to lowered resistance and frequent infections. The occurrence of chronic congestion or night cough, eczema, frequent colds, ear infections, or behavior problems are possible signs of food allergies. They should be investigated to see if this is the case. Avoidance of the offending foods, a rotation diet, or possibly homeopathic treatment will help the body to cope with the physical stresses of viruses and bacteria more efficiently.

Preschoolers and older children may not be the greatest eaters in the world, but if parents limit refined foods, sweets, and junk foods then the result should be a healthy body with a high resistance to infection. Children of all ages develop a sense of values about food. If parents set an example of healthful living and eating, then their children will be more likely to choose healthful foods. This is an important step in the establishment of immune system integrity and a lifelong pattern of wellness. Most children love sweets and these should be limited in all situations. Some children are more sensitive to sugar than others. They may develop symptoms of overactivity, distractibility, and poor self-control after eating sugar. Children often crave foods that stimulate allergic reactions in their bodies, and parents should be alert to these cravings as well as food reactions.

Parents should not underestimate their influence on immune system functioning. The actions that you take can have a direct effect on the immune system. Diet, drugs, medications, and vaccinations all have significant effects. A good diet, avoidance of conventional medications, and the use of natural medicines that stimulate healthy immune system function will provide a good base for a high resistance to infection and prevention of complications of illnesses.

Improved sanitation is one of the most important factors contributing to the decline in incidence of infectious diseases during the past century. Improvements in sanitation and living conditions preceded the development and use of vaccines. Long before the era of antibiotics and specific treatment of infectious diseases, the incidence of pertussis, measles, smallpox, and scarlet fever was decreasing as a direct result of improved hygiene and sanitation practices. These factors are now taken for granted in the United States. When overcrowding and lower standards of living are prevalent in a community, the incidence of infectious diseases and their complications is often significantly higher.

Finally, mental and emotional health provide a key determinant in resistance to infection. Emotional stress is associated with immune system dysfunction, lowered resistance, and more severe forms of infection. The immune system is enhanced in its healthy functions by relaxation, regular rest and sleep, enjoyable activities, and reduction of stress. These factors may be significant for today's children, who have busier schedules and increasing stress from academic demands and parental expectations. We are now in a position to create environments for children which will foster emotional health and decrease stress. If we promote emotional resiliency in children by increasing self-confidence and fulfillment, then a stronger immune system will be the reward. This can be accomplished in many ways. Children thrive when they receive positive reinforcement and praise for their accomplishments and growth. Children want to succeed. Love, attention, and encouragement are parental tools that stimulate a child's well-being. Learning settings that foster exploration, discovery, and creativity will produce inquisitive minds. Strength of spirit and emotional well-being are associated with healthy physical development. Children who feel confident, strong, and happpy are more likely to have an efficient immune system.

PART II:

The Immunizations

The Diseases and their Vaccines

The following sections discuss individual diseases and the vaccines currently recommended by the Center for Disease Control for children in the United States. I present a brief summary of each disease and vaccine and the critical factors surrounding its use. I have included information about disease incidence, vaccine efficacy, and vaccine side effects because these figures are not readily available to the general public. Statistics concerning disease incidence always refer to the United States unless specifically stated otherwise. Each section includes many references to the medical literature because I feel parents should have facts about vaccines, not just opinions and official recommendations. Our knowledge about vaccines is limited, but parents need to be involved in the controversy that this partial picture generates. This technical information may or may not be compelling for you. It is summarized in tables at the end of each section.

There is no question that the incidence of individual diseases has declined, at least in part, because of vaccine administration. But the cost in side effects from the vaccines may be too high for us to tolerate, given our present level of knowledge about the vaccines and disease occurrence. I have included my own recommendations for vaccine use, so parents will know where I stand. Ultimately, the decision about your child rests with you.

29

Tetanus

The preventable disease that parents worry about most is tetanus. This disease is caused by a microorganism that enters the skin through a wound. This condition is in contrast to all the other diseases discussed in this book, which are contracted from other people carrying the organism. Tetanus is potentially fatal, and it strikes otherwise healthy individuals. The repeated exposure of young children to cuts, scrapes, and dirt provides a continual source of anxiety for parents of unvaccinated children. The organism responsible for tetanus is found in soil and the intestinal tracts of farm animals. Any manure-treated soil may be infectious.

The symptoms of tetanus begin with stiffness of muscles; the muscles of the jaw and neck are the first to be involved. In the 24 to 48 hours after onset of the disease, muscle rigidity may be fully developed and involve the trunk and extremities. The neck and back become stiff and arched and the abdomen boardlike. Painful spasms can be produced by the slightest stimulant (noise, touch, light), and it is the spasms of the respiratory muscles that cause asphyxia and death.

The incubation period for tetanus varies from one day to three weeks, although the usual range is one to two weeks. There is no sign of tetanus in the wound itself and usually no symptoms until the muscle stiffness begins. Fever is generally low grade or absent and the senses remain clear.

Treatment for tetanus is drastic. Muscle relaxants, sedatives, antibiotics, immune globulin, and antitoxins are administered. The person is put in a low-stimulus environment, often fed through a stomach tube, and an artificial airway may be required during treatment. There is no effective alternative treatment.

Incidence

Some statistics will help to put the tetanus problem into perspective. Since 1976 there have been less than 100 cases of tetanus per year in the United States (MMWR, 1987). The majority of these cases are people over age 50, and tetanus is now recognized as primarily a disease of older adults in the US. In 1985-1986 only 5 percent of tetanus cases were less than 20 years old (total of 7 cases) (MMWR, 1987). The case-fatality ratio for those individuals less than 50 years old was 5 percent. In other words, only a few cases of tetanus occurred each year in children and these were very rarely fatal. During 1982-1984 a total of 6 tetanus cases occurred in children and adolescents (plus an additional 3 neonatal cases). No deaths occurred among any tetanus cases under 30 years of age (MMWR, 1985). The total case-fatality ratio was 28 percent during 1982-1986. The higher distribution of tetanus cases among the elderly is generally attributed to the low rate of tetanus immunization among this group. Over 95 percent of children entering school since 1980 have received a primary series of tetanus immunizations. By contrast, serosurveys indicate that one-half to two-thirds of persons 60 or older lack protective levels of circulating antitoxin antibody against tetanus (MMWR, 1985). The high percentage of immunized children is at least partially responsible for the low incidence of tetanus in this age group. Just prior to the era of widespread immunization there were approximately 500 cases of tetanus each year.

To summarize this data, young people do not tend to get tetanus, and fatalities are extremely rare. Older people get tetanus more and the case-fatality rate is higher (about 30 percent). Less than 100 cases of tetanus each year is a very low incidence, especially if a large percentage of the older population has no immunity. Tetanus seems to be nearly eliminated from the United States, primarily because of good hygiene and proper wound management. Unlike the contagious diseases, the use of vaccines in some of the population will not help to protect those who are not immunized.

Vaccine administration

The primary series of tetanus toxoid immunization consists of four injections. The first three doses are given at two-month intervals (though the intervals may be longer without forfeiting immunity) and the fourth dose about one year after the third dose. Boosters are recommended at five years old and every ten years thereafter. If a child has had the initial series of shots and recommended boosters, he or she does not need any further shots after injuries. Tetanus toxoid is often combined with other vaccines (e.g. diphtheria and pertussis in DTP), though it can be given alone.

It has been shown that protection from tetanus following adequate immunization lasts for at least twelve years. In people who have had at least two doses of tetanus toxoid previous to an injury, response to an injection of toxoid is rapid and adequate to prevent tetanus.

For individuals who have had less than two previous injections of tetanus toxoid, an injection of Tetanus Immune Globulin, Human (TIG) is administered for serious wounds. This vaccine introduces antibodies directly into the body to fight tetanus bacteria. This is known as passive immunization; the body does not develop its own antibodies. The antibody levels achieved with TIG are sufficient to protect against tetanus.

Vaccine efficacy

There is no question that a series of tetanus toxoid injections is highly effective at preventing tetanus (Edsall, 1959).

This has been documented in several large studies during World War II and with studies of large groups of horses. The fact that all recent tetanus cases in the United States occurred in individuals who had not received the recommended schedule of immunizations provides further evidence that active immunization is extremely effective.

The effectiveness of Tetanus Immune Globulin (TIG) in protecting previously unimmunized individuals at the time of injury is more difficult to document. It is not possible to conduct controlled studies in humans. Judging the efficacy of tetanus immune globulin in the prevention of tetanus must be accomplished by measuring antibody responses after injection and by clinical experience. TIG does raise antibodies in previously nonimmune individuals to levels that indicate adequate protection from tetanus for at least 28 days (McComb and Dwyer, 1963). In addition, the record of tetanus immune globulin in the prevention of fatalities from tetanus is extremely good. Clinical experience with TIG has led to a high level of confidence in the ability to prevent tetanus and death from tetanus when the immune globulin is used in adequate doses within the prescribed interval following injury. There have been rare cases of fatalities in individuals who received tetanus immune globulin soon after injury (Johnson, 1969), but it is generally assumed that one dose of TIG will provide protection.

Vaccine reactions

Tetanus toxoid has been associated with a reaction incidence of 3 to 13 percent (White, W.G. *et al.*, 1983; Relihan, 1969). Side effects include swelling and abscesses at the injection site (Church and Richards, 1985) and allergic reactions after repeated exposure (McComb and Levine, 1961). Hypersensitivity reactions can be quite severe, including fever, abdominal pain, joint pain, weakness, and debility. The long-term side effects are unknown.

Tetanus immune globulin (human) has not been associated with reactions. Since it is a product made from human serum, it may contain infectious material, though this possibility is highly unlikely. All globulin products are tested for contamination by known pathogens such as hepatitis and HIV viruses. The alcohol fractionation process used in the production of TIG is a further safeguard, since this processing destroys such contaminating microorganisms.

TABLE 3

Tetanus Summary

1. Tetanus is a potentially life-threatening disease.

2. Infection occurs through wounds.

3. Incidence of tetanus is 100 cases per year; less than 10 of these cases are under 30 years old, and these cases are rarely fatal.

4. A series of tetanus toxoid injections does provide protection from tetanus for at least 10 years. Tetanus immune globulin protects unimmunized individuals if they receive an injection soon after injury.

5. Immediate vaccine reactions are usually mild and rarely severe. Long-term side effects are unknown.

Recommendations

Parents should decide whether the low risk from possible tetanus exposure warrants giving the vaccine. This is primarily an issue of parental comfort level and likelihood of exposure. A child who lives on a farm or works with horses is more likely to be exposed than one who lives in urban or suburban areas. Parental anxiety about tetanus may be high because the disease progresses rapidly and can attack healthy children. Each parent must make the difficult decision about the tetanus vaccine.

I cannot recommend the tetanus toxoid vaccine for most children because of the unknown risks from long-term effects of the vaccine. This point makes the issues surrounding tetanus obscure. If a child has a high likelihood of exposure or is traveling to a foreign country where sanitation is poor and the incidence of tetanus is higher than the United States, then tetanus vaccine administration should be seriously considered.

Some tetanus vaccine issues are clear. There is no reason to immunize infants because they are extremely unlikely to injure themselves. Delay of immunization may prevent side-effects. A child does not need any protection from tetanus until he or she is old enough to play outdoors and get scrapes and cuts. Children under two years old are not at risk of contracting tetanus.

Some parents may feel that the tetanus vaccine is necessary even if they have decided against giving others. Tetanus toxoid is available as a single vaccine, or combined with diphtheria toxoid, or combined with diphtheria and pertussis. Parents can therefore choose to give the tetanus vaccine alone. Do not allow your child to receive any vaccine you do not want.

Parents can decide to do one of two things:

(1) Give the series of tetanus toxoid injections (preferably after 12 months of age). After the primary series, a child only needs boosters every 10 years, regardless of injuries sustained.

(2) Avoid the routine series and give TIG (Tetanus Immune Globulin, human) only if a child has a serious wound or a deep puncture.

Anyone with a serious wound should receive tetanus immune globulin (TIG) if they have had less than two previous injections of tetanus toxoid. The human immune globulin (TIG) contains tetanus antibodies which will directly attack circulating tetanus bacteria. This will help prevent the multiplication of bacteria and developing infection if it is given within a few days of injury. TIG will not confer lasting immunity to tetanus.

By contrast, tetanus toxoid will not provide adequate protection in previously unimmunized people until the second dose
of the series is given 1 to 2 months after the first. This is too
long a period of time to protect a person from a wound that
has already occurred.

All wounds should be adequately cleansed. This subject
was discussed in an article by Drs. Skudder and McCarrol in
the Journal of the American Medical Association in the 1960s,
when physician encounters with unimmunized people were
more common than today. Their statements and recommendations help to establish guidelines for the treatment of wounds.

> Good wound care is probably the single most important
> factor in the prevention of tetanus in fresh wounds. This
> implies thorough cleansing of the wound and removal of all
> foreign bodies and devitalized [dead] tissue. This is impor-
> tant since the tetanus bacillus is an anaerobic organism and
> can grow only in necrotic tissue which has no blood supply.
> For adequate prophylaxis of tetanus, wounds must be
> divided arbitrarily into those considered tetanus prone and
> non-prone. . . . Any wound containing foreign material or
> devitalized tissue must be considered tetanus prone, as well
> as crushing injuries, deep second and third degree burns,
> [and] any infected wound . . .
> The severity of a wound is not a reliable guide to the
> likelihood of tetanus developing since the disease may arise
> from minor or even unnoticed injuries. Many tetanus prone
> wounds, however, can be converted to non-prone wounds
> by proper cleansing and debridement (Skudder and McCar-
> roll, 1964).

Children who are not immunized should have all wounds
carefully cleansed at home or by a qualified health professional. If a serious wound occurs or there is a question about
the need for tetanus protection, then the advice of a qualified
physician should be sought and the administration of tetanus
immune globulin (TIG) should be considered.

Polio

At its worst, poliomyelitis is a disease that invades the nervous system and produces weakness and flaccid paralysis of the muscles supplied by affected nerves. Polio has probably existed for centuries, but no major epidemics occurred until the end of the nineteenth century. During the period 1900-1930, 80-90 percent of those afflicted with diagnosed polio were under five years of age, and the disease received its name of "infantile paralysis." No epidemics have occurred in the United States since 1954.

In underdeveloped countries where sanitation is poor, polioviruses are widespread. Almost 100 percent of children develop antibodies due to infection in infancy. Paralytic cases are few, the great majority being minor illnesses, and epidemics are unknown. As standards of living change, epidemics can be predicted to occur within a few years. This may be due to lack of general exposure to the virus and sub-sequent greater susceptibility in large numbers of people when virulent strains appear later. Immunization campaigns have also been associated with dramatic increases in polio cases in developing countries.

The polio virus enters the body through the nose or mouth and multiplies in the digestive tract. From there it enters the bloodstream and may then infect nerve cells. Most cases (90-98 percent) of illness associated with poliovirus are either inapparent or characterized by sore throat, headache, nausea, and abdominal pain. It is usually diagnosed as a cold or flu. Paralytic polio begins in the same way and after a few days of minor illness is followed by a few days of well-being. But this is followed by the same symptoms in more severe form, accompanied by stiffness of the back and neck, and muscle pain. Paralysis of the arms and/or legs soon follows. Rarely, paralysis of the muscles of respiration occurs. Return of muscle power begins after a period of days or weeks, and usually reaches its limit in 18 months. After that, any residual paralysis is permanent. Fatalities occur in 5-10 percent of the cases of paralytic polio, usually from respiratory paralysis.

There is no effective specific orthodox treatment for paralytic polio. Homeopaths have treated cases of paralytic polio with reported success, though no studies of treatment effectiveness have been conducted.

Incidence

Wild polio does not exist in the United States at this time. All cases of paralytic polio in this country since 1979 were either caused by the oral vaccine or contracted in a foreign country during travel. During the period 1980-1985, 55 cases of paralytic polio were reported. Of these cases, 51 were caused by the vaccine and 4 occurred in people returning from developing countries (MMWR, 1986).

Vaccine efficacy

Two forms of vaccine are available. The inactivated or killed-virus vaccine, IPV (Salk), is given by injection. It works by producing circulating antibodies only. Booster doses are required as antibody levels decline. The oral live-virus vaccine, OPV (Sabin), produces both intestinal and circulating antibodies, which apparently persist at high levels for years. The oral live-virus vaccine (OPV) replaced the killed vaccine (IPV) in 1962. The oral vaccine was favored because it was easier to administer, it was expected to produce longer-lasting and more complete immunity, and it would produce "herd immunity" in unvaccinated contacts of vaccine recipients.

There is a great deal of controversy concerning the effectiveness of the immunization. Proponents claim the vaccine was responsible for the dramatic decline in polio cases subsequent to the mass immunization campaigns of the late 1950s. Critics suggest that the epidemic just lost its steam. In Great Britain the incidence of death from polio was at its height in 1950. By 1956, when the vaccine campaign was begun, it had already declined by 82 percent. Walene James, in her book *Immunization: The Reality Behind the Myth*, accuses the medical profession of distorting statistics to prove the vaccine's efficacy.

Dr. Bernard Greenberg, a biostatistics expert, was chairman of the Committee on Evaluation and Standards of the American Public Health Association during the 1950s. He testified at a panel discussion that was used as evidence for the congressional hearings on polio vaccine in 1962. During these hearings he elaborated on the problems associated with polio statistics and disputed claims for the vaccine's effectiveness. He attributed the dramatic decline in polio cases to a change in reporting practices by physicians. Less cases were identified as polio after the immunization for very specific reasons. This discussion has relevance to other vaccine experiences as well, and his remarks are therefore quoted at length.

> Prior to 1954 any physician who reported paralytic poliomyelitis was doing his patient a service by way of subsidizing the cost of hospitalization and was being community-minded in reporting a communicable disease. The criterion of diagnosis at that time in most health departments followed the World Health Organization definition: "Spinal paralytic poliomyelitis: signs and symptoms of nonparalytic poliomyelitis with the addition of partial or complete paralysis of one or more muscle groups, detected on two examinations at least 24 hours apart."
>
> Note that "two examinations at least 24 hours apart" was all that was required. Laboratory confirmation and pres-

ence of residual paralysis was not required. In 1955 the
criteria were changed to conform more closely to the definition used in the 1954 field trials: residual paralysis was
determined 10 to 20 days after onset of illness and again 50
to 70 days after onset. . . .

This change in definition meant that in 1955 we started
reporting a new disease, namely, paralytic poliomyelitis
with a longer-lasting paralysis. Furthermore, diagnostic pro-
cedures have continued to be refined. Coxsackie virus infections and aseptic meningitis have been distinguished from
paralytic poliomyelitis. Prior to 1954 large numbers of these
cases   undoubtedly   were   mislabeled   as   paralytic
poliomyelitis. Thus, simply by changes in diagnostic
criteria, the number of paralytic cases was predetermined to
decrease in 1955-1957, whether or not any vaccine was
used. . . .

There is still another reason for the decrease in the
reported paralytic poliomyelitis cases in 1955-57. As a result
of the publicity given the Salk vaccine, the public questioned the possibility of a vaccinated child developing
paralytic poliomyelitis. Whenever such an event occurred,
every effort was made to ascertain whether or not the disease was truly paralytic poliomyelitis. . . . We have been
conditioned today to screen out false positive cases in a way
that was not even imagined prior to 1954.

As a result of these changes in both diagnosis and
diagnostic methods, the rates of paralytic poliomyelitis
plummeted from the early 1950s to a low in 1957 (Intensive
Immunization Programs, Hearings, 1962; p. 96-97).

These factors called into question the claims for polio
vaccine efficacy and the polio vaccine campaign in general.

Vaccine reactions

The oral live-virus polio vaccine is capable of causing
paralytic polio in the vaccine recipient and close contacts. The
person being immunized is more susceptible following the first
dose of live vaccine than after subsequent doses. The risk of
acquiring polio from this vaccine is 1:560,000 for the first dose
(Marcuse, 1989). The risk to household contacts is about 1 per

6 million vaccinees, and 1 per 23 million for community contacts (Nightingale, 1977). The risk of acquiring wild polio is zero.

The injectable "killed" polio vaccine (IPV) does not cause polio. It can cause side effects. These include rare allergic reactions with neurologic symptoms, fevers, and paralysis (JAMA, 1959).

TABLE 4
Polio Summary

1. No wild cases of polio have occurred in the United States since 1979.

2. The vaccines have questionable effectiveness.

3. Oral, live-virus vaccine (OPV) does cause polio in vaccine recipients and contacts.

4. Killed polio vaccine (IPV) has some side effects, but does not cause polio in recipients.

Recommendations

Since the risk of acquiring polio is near zero if a child is not immunized, it seems unjustifiable to risk polio from the live vaccine. The only likely means of exposure to polio are travel to a foreign country, and contact with the feces of another child who has been immunized with the oral vaccine within the previous 6 to 8 weeks. The latter exposure can be minimized by informing daycare providers of the non-immunized status of your child and ensuring that they take proper precautions with handwashing and disposal of soiled diapers of recently immunized children.

If you still have concerns about polio, then the killed vaccine (IPV) is an option. The disadvantage is lower levels of antibody production, more associated reactions, and the

need for boosters to maintain immunity. The recent development of an enhanced-potency inactivated polio vaccine (E-
IPV) has overcome some of the problems associated with the
lower effectiveness of the old vaccine. The 1988 Institute of
Medicine panel on polio vaccine concluded:

> Most parents concerned only for their child's welfare
> and informed about the nature of the alternatives would be
> likely to prefer one of the IPV vaccination strategies. . . .
> [A vaccination schedule] in which two or more doses of
> E-IPV were given prior to OPV would reduce or even elimi-
> nate cases of vaccine-associated paralysis in recipients of
> OPV and in their contacts (Institute of Medicine, 1988).

Vaccine authorities suggest that the oral vaccine is still
needed to produce intestinal immunity and prevent the spread
of polio virus if it is introduced into a community. They
suggest two or more doses of E-IPV followed by OPV at 18
months of age and at entry to elementary school (Institute of
Medicine, 1988). This would reduce the risk of acquiring polio
from the oral vaccine from 1 in 560,000 to 1 in 10.5 million
(Marcuse, 1989). If children receive the oral vaccine, then
non-immunized family members should be immunized as
well.

Pertussis (Whooping Cough)

The vaccine controversy has reached its emotional and political zenith with the publicity generated by pertussis vaccine reactions. Public awareness was fueled by television documentaries, books in the popular press (Coulter & Fisher, 1985), and many magazine articles. Children in Great Britain and Sweden no longer receive the pertussis vaccine, Japan has postponed pertussis immunization until children are two years old, and the United States Congress passed the National Childhood Vaccine Injury Act to provide compensation to parents of children injured by vaccines.

The heightened interest in the pertussis vaccine is associated with the consistent reports of dramatic vaccine reactions and permanent damage suffered by children who have received this vaccine since it was first introduced. Reactions to the vaccine have included fever, persistent crying, encephalitis, epilepsy, retardation, and death. Other neurologic diseases have been associated with the vaccine as well.

Pertussis is an infectious disease of childhood, associated with a specific bacteria. It can sometimes have dramatic and alarming symptoms. The characteristic cough of pertussis usually makes this disease recognizable. The cough comes in paroxysms and is often preceded by a feeling of apprehension or anxiety and tightness in the chest. The cough itself consists of short explosive expirations in rapid succession followed by a long crowing inspiration. During the coughing spell, the child's face may become red or even blue, the eyes bulge, and the tongue protrudes. A number of such paroxysms are sometimes followed by spitting up a mucus plug and vomiting. This will end the attack and the child will rest or appear dazed. Many of these attacks may occur in one day, more frequently at night and in a stuffy room. They may be brought on by physical exertion, crying, and often by eating or drinking. Attacks diminish when the child is concentrating on toys, books, etc. Infants, however, do not always have "whooping" with their cough. The disease usually lasts for at least 6 weeks regardless of treatment. Complications of pertussis may include cerebral hemorrhage, convulsions and brain damage, pneumonia, emphysema, or collapsed lung. Deaths are usually due to complicating respiratory infection. Pneumonia is the most frequent cause of death in children under three years of age.

Standard treatment with antibiotics may help reduce the period of contagion to others and prevent complications. Pertussis immune globulin may help shorten the illness and prevent complications and deaths in children under two years of age. Homeopathic treatment has been used extensively in the past, and one recent study suggests there may be a beneficial effect from homeopathy on pertussis (English, 1987b). This survey followed children who received a homeopathic preventive for pertussis and subsequently did contract the disease and were then treated homeopathically. The results of this survey suggested that the group of children treated with homeopathy experienced relatively mild cases of pertussis, compared to children who received antibiotic treatment. The author of this study acknowledges that the number of children followed was too small to make any definitive conclusions about the efficacy of homeopathy in the treatment of pertussis.

Incidence

Pertussis still occurs with regularity as a common childhood disease. Prior to 1940, it was estimated that 95 percent of all individuals had some form of pertussis during their life. The incidence of pertussis has declined from at least 100 reported cases per 100,000 population during the period 1930-1945 to an average of 1 per 100,000 population during 1973-1985. There are now several thousand cases per year. Most occur during childhood. During 1976-1985 there were 4 to 11 reported deaths per year associated with pertussis.

Vaccine efficacy

The most reliable studies of vaccine efficacy involve vaccinated children living in a house with someone who has contracted the disease. These types of studies have shown a variation in vaccine efficacy of 63 to 91 percent (Cherry *et al.*, 1988). One study showed an efficacy of 80 percent 3 years after the last dose, 50 percent between 4 and 7 years, and none after 12 years (Lambert, 1965). This is not a very high level of efficacy. In other words, the vaccine may not work in a large percentage of children.

Vaccine reactions

Several large studies have been conducted to investigate pertussis vaccine side effects because of the consistent publicity generated by case reports of severe reactions since the vaccine was introduced. Epidemiologists have difficulty attributing apparent reactions to the pertussis vaccine for several reasons. The most problematic is that fevers, seizures, and sudden unexplained death (SIDS) all occur during the first year of life in the unvaccinated as well as the vaccinated. Since 95 percent of children in the United States are vaccinated, it is difficult (and probably unethical) to find a placebo control group.

The most comprehensive pertussis study was conducted in Los Angeles during 1978-1979, the UCLA study (Cody *et al.*, 1981). Children who received the DTP vaccine were compared to those who received the DT vaccine. Reactions that occurred during the first 48 hours after vaccine administration were recorded. The most serious criticism of the UCLA study and other similar studies is that the vaccine may cause delayed reactions not apparent within the first two days. Delayed reactions are difficult to distinguish from the background occurrence of these problems. Dr. Harris Coulter, medical historian and author of two books on vaccine damage, has postulated that a wide array of neurologic problems can be attributed to these delayed or initially imperceptible reactions. In fact, he says, these represent an allergic encephalitis which is only diagnosed when effects are observed later in life.

> Severe neurologic sequelae may also occur after vaccination in the absence of an acute reaction. When the baby reacts to a DPT shot with "a slight fever and fussiness for a few days," this may be, and often is, a case of encephalitis which is quite capable of causing even quite severe long-term neurologic consequences. . . . Any researcher who ignores or rejects the possibility that vaccination can cause the most serious neurologic disorders in the absence of a marked acute reaction will have to find grounds for distinguishing post-vaccinal encephalitis from encephalitis due to other causes (Coulter, 1990).

The UCLA study data show that 50 percent of vaccinees developed fever, 34 percent irritability, 35 percent had crying episodes, and 40 percent had localized inflammation. The more significant major reactions included 3 percent of children who had persistent crying, and 31 percent with excessive sleepiness (compared to 14 percent in the DT controls). The occurrence of seizures could not be statistically verified because of the small numbers of children (16,536 immunizations in the total study). A study with larger numbers did find a significant difference in seizure occurrence when 134,000 children receiving DTP were compared to 133,000 DT recipients (Pollock & Morris, 1983). The authors of this study questioned whether these reactions were overreported by participating physicians because of the adverse publicity concerning the pertussis vaccine.

Even more controversy surrounds the relationship of permanent neurologic damage (encephalopathy and retardation) to the pertussis vaccine. The typical case involves an initial seizure after the vaccine's administration, followed by recurrent seizures after a few days or weeks. Then mental and motor retardation become apparent over the ensuing months (Cherry *et al.*, 1988). The most reliable study conducted to investigate neurologic disorders after DTP vaccine was carried out in England, Wales, and Scotland during 1976-1979, the National Childhood Encephalopathy Study (NCES) (Alderslade *et al.*, 1981). This case-control study sought to find a risk factor for vaccine reaction by examining all cases of neurologic disease and comparing those cases to a control group. Only hospitalized cases were examined. DTP immunization had occurred significantly more frequently within the previous 72-hour and the seven-day period in the children with neurologic illness than in the controls. The estimated risk of serious neurologic disorder within seven days after DTP was 1:110,000 immunizations, and the estimated risk of occurrence of persistent neurologic damage 1 year later was 1:310,000. These figures have been assailed by parties on both sides of the controversy. Through an analysis of the data, Dr. James Cherry of UCLA and his colleagues determined that the temporal association of DTP with neurologic disease merely indicates that the vaccine has brought out symptoms that would have occurred anyway.

Dr. Harris Coulter and his co-author, Barbara Loe Fisher, insist that these figures grossly underestimate the true extent of damage caused by the pertussis vaccine, because the criteria for symptom occurrence are much too limited (Coulter & Fisher, 1985). In fact, Coulter would attribute a much larger number of "soft" neurodevelopmental symptoms (learning disorders, attention deficits, and behavior problems) to the vaccine. He suggests that delayed vaccine reactions are often responsible for these permanent disabilities (Coulter, 1990).

The relationship of pertussis vaccine to deaths is even more controversial. Three studies have found a temporal association between infant deaths and DTP immunization (Baraff *et al.*, 1983; Torch 1982; Waler *et al.*, 1987). In Waler's case-control study the relative risk for SIDS (sudden infant death syndrome) within 3 days of immunization was 7.3, a very significant risk. This included 4 of the 29 SIDS cases reviewed. Four other studies found no significant association. Not unexpectedly, the American Academy of Pediatrics Task Force on Pertussis concluded that there is no convincing evidence for a causative role for DTP immunization in SIDS in their review of these 7 studies (Cherry *et al.*, 1988).

Regardless of these controversies it is clear that the pertussis vaccine is dangerous. Parents must ultimately decide whether they want to risk the side effects of immunization. It is parents who are responsible for the passage of the vaccine compensation law. Parents initiated the lawsuits which have consistently resulted in monetary awards for vaccine damage. And this pressure has caused the present situation where most pharmaceutical manufacturers have stopped producing DTP vaccine.

TABLE 5

Pertussis Summary

1. The vaccine is associated with severe reactions including encephalitis, seizures, brain damage, and deaths.

2. The disease itself has these same risks, though the incidence of pertussis is now low in the United States.

3. The vaccine has limited efficacy.

4. The disease can be treated with homeopathic medications, antibiotics, and immune globulin.

Recommendations

I advise against the pertussis vaccine because of the significant risk from the shot, and because homeopathy is able to provide treatment for whooping cough when it occurs (English, 1987b). Before anyone gives their child a pertussis shot, I recommend that they read the case descriptions in Coulter and Fisher's book. No amount of controversial statistics can compare to the harrowing and heart-wrenching accounts of parents with vaccine-injured children.

Diphtheria

Diphtheria is an acute infectious disease caused by a bacteria. The disease is characterized by a sore throat and development of a membrane that may cover the throat. It can become a dangerous disease if this membrane makes it difficult or impossible to breathe. Complications of diphtheria include (1) myocarditis (infection within the heart), which can lead to heart failure, and (2) transitory paralysis of the limbs, muscles of respiration (sometimes causing death), or muscles of the throat or eye. The incubation period is two to four days.

Incidence

Diphtheria is an extremely rare disease. The number of cases has steadily declined during the past century. For example, between 1900 and 1920 the mortality rate from diphtheria declined by 50 percent (Mortimer, 1978). This preceded the immunization era. During the 1940s, reported diphtheria cases numbered 15,000 to 30,000 per year in the United States. By the 1960s the number of cases declined to 200 to 1,000 per year. And in the 1980s there were 0 to 5 cases per year.

Vaccine efficacy

There is some question about the effectiveness of diphtheria vaccine. A classic situation occurred in Germany during World War II. When diphtheria immunization was made mandatory there was a 17 percent increase in the number of cases and a 600 percent rise in the number of deaths from diphtheria. When the vaccine was stopped at the end of the war, the incidence of diphtheria dramatically declined, despite the poor living conditions and malnutrition. During an epidemic of diphtheria in Chicago during 1969, 25 percent of the cases had been fully immunized, and an additional 12 percent showed serologic evidence of full immunity, though they had received less than the full series of shots (Mendelsohn, 1978).

TABLE 6
Diphtheria Summary

1. Diphtheria is a potentially serious disease but extremely rare in the United States, with an incidence of less than 5 cases per year.

2. The vaccine has questionable effectiveness.

3. Long-term effects of the vaccine are unknown.

Recommendations

At the present time this vaccine seems unnecessary due to the low incidence of disease and questionable vaccine efficacy.

Measles, Mumps, and Rubella

Immunization for these diseases is usually given as a single shot of combined live viruses (the MMR vaccine) at 15 months of age or older. Mass immunization of children for mumps, measles, and rubella has resulted in a shift in the pattern of these diseases. The age distribution has changed significantly since the vaccines were introduced in the 1960s. Now these are increasingly becoming diseases of adolescents and young adults. This is a problem since the diseases themselves cause more complications in this older population. Secondly, the vaccines seem to have caused atypical forms of the diseases to appear. It should also be remembered that the natural occurrence of each of these viral diseases generally confers permanent immunity against subsequent attacks.

Measles

Measles was a common disease of childhood prior to the widespread use of measles vaccine. The disease is transmitted by a virus, which is highly contagious. The symptoms of measles are cold symptoms, cough, irritated eyes, and high fever, with the appearance of a rash on the fourth day of illness. The symptoms, including the rash, reach a climax on about the sixth day and then subside in a few days. Measles occasionally sets the stage for other diseases. These complications include ear infections, pneumonia, infection of lymph nodes, and encephalitis, but they are not common. In the past, deaths from measles were not uncommon during epidemics. Now the disease has become milder and deaths are rare. Measles is usually a self-limited disease. Encephalitis is reported to occur in one out of 1,000 cases, though this figure is probably exaggerated. Of these encephalitis cases, 25 to 30 percent show manifestations of brain damage.

Orthodox medicine has no specific treatment for measles or measles-associated encephalitis. Homeopaths feel confident about their ability to prevent complications, though no efficacy studies have been conducted.

Incidence

Measles was contracted by most children prior to vaccine licensure. Since the licensing of measles vaccine in 1963, the

incidence of measles has declined to less than 2 percent of
previous levels (Markowitz *et al.*, 1989). Recently, incidence
has declined from an average of 40,000 reported cases per year
in the 1970s to an average of 3,000 per year in the 1980s.

Vaccine efficacy

The vaccine has apparently resulted in a dramatic decline
in measles cases. In the light of these promising statistics, a
national goal was set to eliminate measles by 1982. Not-
withstanding these hopes, reports of epidemics in fully vaccinated populations have appeared periodically and consistently
since the vaccine's introduction (Shasby *et al.*, 1977; Weiner
et al., 1977; Hull *et al.*, 1985). A typical example was reported
by Dr. Tracy Gustafson and colleagues in the *New England
Journal of Medicine*. During the spring of 1985 a measles outbreak occurred in two fully immunized secondary school populations (greater than 99 percent of students immunized). On
serologic testing, 95 percent of students showed immunity to
measles. The epidemic occurred in the remaining 5 percent,
all of whom had been "adequately" vaccinated (Gustafson *et
al.*, 1987). Some authors have postulated that a waning
immunity over time is responsible for these outbreaks among
older children (Shasby *et al.*, 1977). Others blame primary
vaccine failure. In any case, the public health goal of eradicat-
ing measles in the United States by 1982 was not met, despite
rigorous vaccine programs. Gustafson concludes that such a
goal is impossible to meet.

Measles cases now consistently occur in the vaccinated.
A review of measles outbreaks in the United States during
1985-1986 revealed that a median of 60 percent of cases in
school-age children occurred in vaccinated individuals (Markowitz *et al.*, 1989). Similarly, a review of 1600 cases of
measles in Quebec, Canada, between January and May 1989
showed that 58 percent of school-age cases had been previously vaccinated (MMWR, 1989a). In states with comprehensive (kindergarten through 12th grade) immunization require-

ments, between 61 and 90 percent of measles cases occur in persons who were appropriately vaccinated (Markowitz *et al.*, 1989).

The official response to measles vaccine failure and epidemics has varied. Within the first ten years after widespread immunization, the vaccine failures prompted public health authorities to repeatedly raise the recommended age for immunization. In 1969 the age for vaccine administration was raised to 12 months or older (Albrecht *et al.*, 1977). Because of continued vaccine failure, the age for administration was subsequently raised to 15 months (MMWR, 1989b). During 1988, an epidemic in Los Angeles prompted a reconsideration of vaccine recommendations when statistics showed that 38 percent of cases were less than 16 months old (MMWR, 1989c). The age for vaccine administration was then lowered again to 9 months in areas with recurrent measles transmission (MMWR, 1989d). These children would then require revaccination at 15 months.

The fact that a large percentage of measles cases occurs in school-age children and adolescents has caused a reassessment of measles vaccination policy. A two-dose measles vaccine schedule is now recommended, both doses in the form of MMR. The first dose is given at 15 months of age or later. The second dose of vaccine is intended to overcome the problems with primary vaccine failure and to reinforce waning immunity. The American Academy of Pediatrics recommends this dose at 11 or 12 years of age (Committee on Infectious Diseases, 1989). The Center for Disease Control recommends this second dose at entry to kindergarten or first grade, 4-6 years of age (MMWR, 1989i). Neither of these policies has been evaluated in any studies.

Vaccine reactions

Serious nervous system and other reactions to measles vaccine have been repeatedly reported in the medical literature. These reactions include encephalitis (Fenichel, 1982; White,

F., 1983), retinopathy and blindness (Marshall *et al.*, 1985), and seizures, Guillain-Barré syndrome (muscle paralysis and sensory nerve deficits), and subacute sclerosing panencephalitis.

The following case of eye damage caused by the measles vaccine was reported by Dr. Gary Marshall and colleagues in the journal *Pediatrics*.

> A 16-month-old baby girl . . . had been previously healthy and developmentally normal. . . . In September 1983, 14 days after measles, mumps, and rubella vaccination, she had subjective fever, cough, conjunctival injection, and a generalized macular erythematous rash. Two days later, the majority of these symptoms abated, but the conjunctival injection worsened, her pupils became dilated, and she began walking into objects. . . . On admission to the hospital, examination revealed a vigorous toddler who would not reach for objects and had only minimal light perception. Ophthalmologic examination showed a diffuse chorioretinitis with perivascular retinal edema, mild papilledema, and a stellate macular configuration. . . . Repeat fundoscopic [eye] examination several days later demonstrated evolution into a "salt and pepper" pigmentary pattern distributed radially along the retinal veins. These changes were most consistent with measles retinopathy. . . . On follow-up examination 7 months later, her visual acuity had improved; she was able to ambulate freely but still sat close to the television set and held objects close to her face. Fundoscopic examination revealed macular scarring (Marshall *et al.*, 1985).

A disturbing syndrome of atypical measles has occurred in children previously immunized. This consists of an illness with exaggerated rash, muscle weakness, peripheral edema, and severe abdominal pain with persistent vomiting (Cherry *et al.*, 1972). These reactions have occurred rarely following the immunization as well (St. Geme, 1976).

Dr. Richard Moskowitz has proposed a possible mechanism for long-term sequelae of measles and other live-virus vaccines. Various viruses, including measles, are capable of stimulating autoimmune responses if they are stored within the body's own cells over long periods of time. He postulates that a similar mechanism may occur following the measles live-virus vaccine.

In the case of the attenuated measles virus, it is not difficult to imagine that introducing it directly into the blood would continue to provoke an antibody response for a considerable period of time, which is doubtless the whole point of giving the vaccine; but that eventually, as the virus succeeded in attaining a state of latency within the cell, the antibody response would wane, both because circulating antibodies cannot normally cross the cell membrane, and because they are also powerful immunosuppressive agents in their own right.

The effect of circulating antibody will thereafter be mainly to keep the virus *within* the cell, i.e. to continue to prevent any acute inflammatory response, until eventually, perhaps under circumstances of accumulated stress or emergency, this precarious balance breaks down, antibodies begin to be produced in large quantities against the cells themselves, and frank auto-immune phenomena of necrosis and tissue destruction supervene (Moskowitz, 1983).

TABLE 7
Measles Summary

---

1. Measles has historically been a common childhood disease with rare complications.

2. Mass immunization has resulted in a dramatic decline in measles incidence, but outbreaks now occur in older populations.

3. The vaccine is associated with serious immediate side effects and unknown long-term reactions.

Recommendations

Parents must decide whether they are willing to risk the known and unknown side effects from the measles vaccine in order to prevent the rare complications of measles. I do not recommend the measles vaccine because of the risk from the vaccine and unknown long-term effects of both the vaccine and waning immunity.

Mumps

Mumps was a common and very mild disease of childhood that was not even noticed in 30 percent of cases prior to widespread vaccine use. The illness begins with fever, headache, and tiredness. Within 24 hours the child complains of earache near the lobe of the ear. The next day the salivary gland in front of the ear becomes swollen. Within one to six days the illness runs its course.

Infection of the testicles, ovaries, and other organs are not unusual, but occur much more commonly in adults. Infection of the testicle occurs in 20 to 30 percent of mumps cases in adolescent or adult males (Philip *et al.*, 1959). Sterility following such an illness is extremely rare. Encephalitis occurs in as many as five cases per 1,000 reported mumps cases. Deaths from mumps are rare, but much more likely to occur in adults; about half of mumps-associated deaths have been in persons over 20 years old (MMWR, 1989g).

Incidence and Vaccine Efficacy

A live mumps virus vaccine was licensed in 1967 and recommended for routine use in 1977. It apparently resulted in a decline in the incidence of mumps cases. But a recent resurgence in mumps cases has caused a reevaluation of the previous optimistic vaccine success reports. The number of mumps cases had decreased during the early 1980s to 3,000 to 5,000 cases per year, a dramatic decline from the 100,000 cases per year of the early 1970s. However, during 1986, 7,800 cases occurred, and during 1987 there were nearly 13,000 reported mumps cases.

The most disturbing factor in these statistics is the shift in mumps cases to older age groups who are much more susceptible to the complications of testicular and ovarian infection. During the period 1967-1971 the annual average of cases in persons ≥15 years of age was 8.3 percent; this age group accounted for 38.3 percent of cases in 1987. This represents a greater than eightfold increase (MMWR, 1989e). Although we are assured that the risk to adolescents is still less than in the pre-vaccine era, this trend is disconcerting. It is thought that the rise in cases among adolescents is due to lack of immunization in children born between 1967 and 1977 and not to waning immunity in persons vaccinated previously (Cochi, 1988). Nonetheless, this shift to older populations is worrisome. Mumps in young children is a mild, benign disease. In adolescents and adults it is a disease associated with more complications. The response among public health authorities is to revaccinate during middle childhood or adolescence.

The efficacy of mumps vaccine has ranged from 75 to 95 percent in various studies.

Vaccine Reactions

The mumps vaccine is associated with side effects similar to the measles vaccine. It has been associated with fevers, seizures, encephalitis, and severe, atypical mumps disease.

Recommendations

Use of the mumps vaccine, which has been associated with serious side effects, seems unjustifiable. Administering the vaccine during adolescence may just prolong the problem of waning immunity and shift the disease and its complications to an even older population.

TABLE 8
Mumps Summary

1. Mumps is generally a benign disease of children.

2. Mumps has increasingly become a disease of adolescents and adults since the widespread use of the vaccine.

3. Complications occur much more frequently in adults.

4. The vaccine has associated side effects and unknown long-term effects.

Rubella (German Measles)

Rubella is a mild childhood illness that consists of fever, rash and tiredness lasting for a few days. It has no serious complications except in very rare instances.

The purpose of immunization is to prevent pregnant women from contracting rubella, since abortion, stillbirths and deformities can result from illness during the first three months of pregnancy. Between 20 and 50 percent of babies born to women who contract rubella during pregnancy will have birth defects (eye defects, deafness, mental retardation). This vaccine is unique in that children are immunized to interrupt circulation of the virus and reduce the risk of exposure to susceptible pregnant women.

Prevention of rubella using the live virus vaccine can be accomplished in one of two ways: (1) immunize susceptible women of child-bearing age, or (2) immunize preschool and school-age children to prevent disease transmission. The question has persistently arisen whether the rubella vaccine should be given to children or to susceptible adolescent and adult women, with many experts on both sides of this controversy. Drs. Otto Sieber and Vincent Fulginiti, recognized vaccine experts, argued against routine immunization of children (Fulginiti, 1976; Sieber & Fulginiti, 1977). When reports appeared that antibody titers decreased after childhood rubella immunization, they stated, "one might argue that immunization of adolescents or adults might be a more appropriate strategy than our current emphasis upon immunization of infants. . . ." If the protective effect of the vaccine decreases over time, then a girl who is immunized during childhood may become susceptible once again as an adult. If the vaccine has significant side effects, then vaccinated children could be needlessly exposed to this risk. Both of these factors argue against the use of rubella vaccine in children.

Another reason for immunization of susceptible adult women rather than children was put forward by Dr. Stephen Schoenbaum and colleagues in 1975 in the *Journal of the American Medical Association*. They discovered that children may not be the major source of rubella spread to pregnant women. They tested a hypothesis.

> If children were an important source of contagion for pregnant women, it should be reflected by one of the following: First, the percentage of women with detectable antibody titers, signifying previous experience with rubella, should rise with increasing parity [number of children born to a woman] more than one would expect on the basis of age alone. Second, the incidence of rubella among susceptible pregnant women should increase with increasing parity and should be reflected by an increasing frequency of babies with rubella syndrome among children born of later pregnancies.

In other words, mothers should show evidence of more exposure to rubella than other women. Their study found the opposite to be true.

> To summarize the serologic data, there was no evidence of a decrease in susceptibility with increasing parity. These data, therefore, offer no support for the presumption that the number of susceptible adult women materially decreases after the first pregnancy. . . . This finding is consistent with the concept that most persons who contract rubella as adults do so through contact with other adults (Schoenbaum *et al.*, 1975).

If children are not the primary source of infection for pregnant women, then children should not be targeted for prevention. They come to the logical conclusion. "We . . . would prefer the alternative policy of selectively and efficiently vaccinating adolescent girls."

Incidence

The incidence of rubella and congenital rubella syndrome has declined dramatically since the vaccine was licensed in 1969. Previous levels of 20,000 to 60,000 reported cases of rubella per year have declined to several hundred per year in the 1980s. During 1988, 221 cases of rubella were reported. In 1987, 3 indigenous cases of congenital rubella syndrome were reported and only 1 was reported in 1988 (MMWR, 1989f).

Vaccine efficacy

The protective effect of rubella vaccine has been estimated as 77 percent in one study (Hough *et al.*, 1979). A continuing concern is the gradual reduction in an individual's antibody titer following rubella immunization. The effectiveness of the vaccine may decrease so that women who were not susceptible as children become susceptible again as adults. In fact, the disease has shifted to older age groups. During the three-year period before vaccine licensure (1966-1968), 23 percent of rubella cases occurred among persons ≥ 15 years of age. In 1987, 48 percent of cases occurred in persons ≥ 15 years old (MMWR, 1989f). Serologic surveys of postpubertal populations have found that rates of rubella susceptibility are comparable to the prevaccine years (10 to 20 percent lack evidence of immunity) (Crowder *et al.*, 1987; Bart *et al.* 1985). The proposed solution to this problem of shifting age occurrence has again been to revaccinate susceptible women of childbearing age.

Vaccine reactions

Side effects of the rubella vaccine include encephalitis-type symptoms, meningitis, and the Guillain-Barré syndrome (muscle paralysis and sensory nerve deficits). In addition, at least 12 to 20 percent of women develop arthritis symptoms after receiving the vaccine. These may begin several weeks after the administration of vaccine (Fulginiti, 1976). They may persist for weeks, months, or years. In some cases, women develop rheumatoid arthritis which continues throughout their lives.

The following case was reported by Dr. J. Richard Gunderman in the *American Journal of Diseases of Children.*

A 20-month-old white boy was well until ten days after inoculation with the combined mumps-rubella vaccine. Initial complaints were the inability to stand on the left leg and pain in all extremities. The weakness progressed to include both legs and ascended to involve all extremities. . . . Examination revealed an apprehensive child with a complete flaccid paralysis of all extremities and inability to hold his head up. The patient had marked soft tissue tenderness of all extremities. Neurologic evaluation revealed no muscle stretch reflexes. . . . Over a three-month period he completely recovered all motor functions (Gunderman, 1973).

This case is similar to other descriptions of weakness or paralysis of extremities, loss of sensation, and difficulty walking in other children who reacted to the rubella vaccine (Kilroy, 1970; Gilmartin *et al.*, 1972).

Recommendations

Parents have three options: avoid the vaccine entirely, immunize their child against rubella, or test girls for antibodies at adolescence or before considering pregnancy and decide whether to immunize then. Since a child's health is not compromised by contracting rubella, there is no advantage to the child from vaccination. Every adolescent girl and woman of

---

TABLE 9
Rubella Summary

---

1. Rubella is a mild disease of childhood which requires no treatment.

2. A woman who contracts rubella during the first three months of pregnancy risks abortion, miscarriage, or birth defects in her child.

3. Rubella incidence has shifted to older age groups since widespread immunization.

4. Rubella vaccine is associated with significant side effects, including arthritis and central nervous system disorders.

---

childbearing age should have a blood test for immunity to rubella. If they do not have evidence of immunity, then they should decide whether they wish to have the vaccine. Susceptible women who decline the vaccine should attempt to avoid exposure to children with colds, fevers, and rashes during the first three months of pregnancy. Again, the consideration is whether the possible side effects of the vaccine are worth prevention of problems during pregnancy. Avoidance of the vaccine during childhood will eliminate the risk of untoward vaccine reactions in your child.

Hemophilus Influenzae Type B (Hib) Meningitis

A relative newcomer to the vaccine field is the *Hemophilus influenzae* b (Hib) vaccine to prevent meningitis. The purified polysaccharide form of the vaccine (PRP) was licensed in 1985. The conjugate form of this vaccine (PRP-D or HbOC) is now recommended for all children 18 months of age or older. The polysaccharide form of the vaccine (PRP) was not effective in children under 24 months old, and these children represent 80 percent of Hib meningitis cases (Ward, 1987). If the PRP form of the vaccine is joined to a protein carrier (in this case diphtheria toxoid), then the vaccine is more effective in young children. This "conjugate" form is now used in the United States. This vaccine is continually being tested on younger children who are more susceptible to Hib meningitis (Eskola *et al.*, 1987). Few large-scale studies have been completed, but the vaccine will probably be recommended for children less than 18 months in the near future.

Meningitis in children often begins with flulike symptoms including fever, headache, nausea and vomiting, tiredness, and irritability. This may be followed by a change in alertness, stiff neck, and seizures. Between 20 and 30 percent of children with bacterial meningitis have seizures. Arthritis, pericarditis, and pneumonia are common complications (Kaplan & Fishman, 1988). Disease of sudden onset with rapid progression is usually associated with a different bacteria, *Neisseria meningitidis*, which has a much higher risk of death . A sudden change in level of alertness or severe headache in children is cause for concern. Mortality from Hib meningitis is 3 to 8 percent (Sell, 1987). Sensorineural (permanent) hearing loss occurs in approximately 10 percent of meningitis cases (Dodge *et al.*, 1984), though this is most common with pneumococcal meningitis. Appropriate treatment of Hib meningitis includes the use of a cephalosporin (or other) antibiotic administered intravenously.

Several studies have observed long-term cognitive effects of previous *Hemophilus influenzae* meningitis on children. Most recent studies have found no differences in IQ scores or academic success of meningitis patients compared to their sibling controls (Tejani *et al.*, 1982; Feldman & Michaels, 1988; R.D. Feigin and P.R. Dodge, unpublished data). But several previously conducted studies did find that learning disabilities, reading problems, and lower IQ scores occurred more frequently in postmeningitic children compared to randomly selected, peer-group controls (Sell *et al.*, 1972; Pate, 1972). This may indicate that Hib meningitis is associated with learning problems, but the validity of this association is still in question.

Incidence

The estimated incidence of Hib meningitis is 8,000 to 15,000 cases per year. Incidence has increased over the past three decades. Some observers associate this increase with the administration of other immunizations and their apparent ability to impair immune system resistance. Although this link has not been proven, the tendency of vaccines to cause neurologic complications has raised suspicions that central nervous system infections occur more frequently as a direct result of DTP and measles vaccine (Coulter, 1990).

Approximately 1 in 350 children younger than 5 years of age develops Hib meningitis (Sell, 1987). Children under 6 months are protected by maternal antibodies, and breastfeeding reduces incidence. The peak incidence of meningitis occurs in children 6 to 7 months of age. The attack rate decreases rapidly with increasing age. Fifty percent of cases occur in infants under 1 year of age. Only 25 to 30 percent of cases occur in children over 18 months old (Broome, 1987). If the vaccine is given only to children over 18 months old, then the majority of potential cases will not be targeted for vaccine.

Vaccine efficacy

In one study, 90 percent of children vaccinated with the conjugate vaccine responded with antibody levels considered to be protective, but only 60 percent produced levels of antibody indicating long-term protection (Berkowitz *et al.*, 1987). The efficacy of the conjugate vaccine has not been determined in field trials (MMWR, 1988).

The effectiveness of the conjugate vaccine was called into question by a case-control study conducted by Dr. Michael Osterholm in Minnesota, published in the *Journal of the American Medical Association*. He found that 41 percent of cases occurred in vaccinated children. The vaccine's protective efficacy was minus 58 percent. In other words, children were much more likely to get the disease if they had received the vaccine (Osterholm *et al.*, 1988). Apparently the vaccine had lowered their resistance and created an environment that encouraged spread of the disease to the nervous system. This is precisely what one would predict if the vaccines do suppress immune system function.

The original polysaccharide form of the vaccine had limited success, as documented in case control studies. Vaccine efficacy ranged from 41 percent to 88 percent in the various studies. An active surveillance study which included a population of two and a half million children under five years of age identified 1,444 cases of invasive *H influenzae* disease. Vaccine efficacy in this group was found to be 62 percent compared to controls. Again a much lower figure than expected by researchers (Harrison *et al.*, 1989).

Vaccine reactions

The *Hemophilus* vaccine is associated with many reactions. Dr. Julie Milstien and colleagues reviewed 152 spontaneous reports of vaccine reactions submitted to the FDA during the first year of vaccine availability, 1985-1986 (Milstien *et al.*, 1987). Serious reactions included convulsions (with and without fever), anaphylactoid allergic reactions, serum sickness-like reactions (joint pain, rashes, and edema), and one death within 4 hours of vaccination. In addition to the reported reactions, there were 63 reports of proven *H influenzae* type b invasive disease that occurred soon after the immunization. These were considered vaccine failures, though they may have been reactions.

TABLE 10

***Hemophilus influenzae* b (Hib) Meningitis Summary**

1. Meningitis is a potentially life-threatening disease and long term sequelae (hearing loss, learning problems) do occur.

2. Most cases of Hib meningitis occur in children under 18 months old, prior to the age vaccine is recommended.

3. The vaccine's ability to prevent meningitis has not been determined.

4. Serious vaccine-associated reactions have been reported.

Recommendations

The vaccine for meningitis has too many unclear aspects. Efficacy is questionable, the frequency of side effects is unknown, and long-term side effects could not be discovered yet for a vaccine recently licensed in 1985. Parents need to decide whether they are willing to risk the possible side effects of a vaccine which is questionably effective, experimental, and not targeted at the population of children under 18 months who are most at risk. I do not recommend its use in normal children.

New Vaccines

The medical profession and drug manufacturers continually develop new vaccines for childhood illness. Research studies are done and eventually the vaccines are licensed for widespread use. Cost analyses determine whether the price of vaccine is worth the prevention of disease and the risk of side effects. Debate on this subject occurs and the FDA decides to license the new vaccine for widespread use. Only then will the millions of dollars invested by drug companies in research and development be recouped many times over in the form of profits.

After a period of time during which large numbers of children are vaccinated, the side effects of each vaccine begin to appear. Hundreds of thousands of children must be vaccinated before these adverse effects appear because vaccine reactions often go unreported, and it is often difficult to attribute late effects to a vaccine. The use of new vaccines is an experiment on healthy children.

No research is done on the long-term effects of vaccines before licensure because drug companies must market their product as quickly as possible. They cannot wait for a thirty-year study. They have little interest in discovering side effects or generating negative data about their vaccines. The impetus to discover these comes from parents of vaccine-injured children and journalists sympathetic to their stories. The medical profession is quick to adopt new vaccines and is generally disinterested in their problems. Foot-dragging, delayed responses to problems with vaccines, and suppression of information are the typical official stances of the medical profession when questions of vaccine safety arise. This course of events has been well documented in Coulter and Fisher's exposé of the pertussis vaccine catastrophe (Coulter and Fisher, 1984). The United States Government was compelled to step in and rescue drug companies from the ruinous lawsuits brought against them by dismayed and angry parents of children damaged by the pertussis vaccine. Financial investments of drug companies and the vaccine industry dictate the direction of research on immunization policy. Their interests lie in promotion of vaccines, not investigation of side effects.

Despite the history of serious vaccine side effects, which includes polio caused by the oral vaccine, deaths and brain damage caused by DTP, and the many problems of live measles and mumps vaccines, drug companies and the medical profession persist in the development and rush to market of new vaccines. Few studies and little experience precede licensure of these new products. Hemophilus, chickenpox, and pneumococcal vaccines are the most recent experiments conducted on America's children.

Varicella (Chickenpox)

Chickenpox is universally recognized as a mild and benign disease of childhood. Almost all children are infected at some time and develop permanent immunity from the disease. The disease is caused by the varicella-zoster virus, a member of the herpesvirus family. The symptoms of chickenpox usually include a fever and runny nose, followed by the appearance of the typical eruption. These are small, flat, pink areas which soon fill with a clear fluid and then open and crust over within 2-3 days. They appear in crops and persist as active lesions for a week. During this time children are usually uncomfortable and itching, especially if they have many eruptions or if these occur on mucus membranes. The disease usually ends uneventfully after a week. Treatment is directed at making children comfortable. Homeopathic treatment may be helpful for the itching and other bothersome symptoms.

Disease Complications

Complications of chickenpox include secondary infections of the skin and neurologic disease. Encephalitis occurs infrequently in children, once in every 4,000 to 10,000 chickenpox cases. Many of these cases are mild, and hospitalization is required once in every 10,000 to 15,000 cases (Guess *et al.*, 1986). The incidence of encephalitis and associated deaths has been decreasing. An average of 58 cases of encephalitis per year was reported between 1972 and 1979. This was reduced to an average of only 28 cases reported between 1980 and 1983 (Preblud, 1986). Reye syndrome, a dangerous encephalopathy characterized by convulsions and coma, is another rare complication of chickenpox. Its incidence has declined dramatically in recent years as well. The recent avoidance of aspirin during chickenpox illnesses may be responsible for the reduction in Reye syndrome. Deaths from chickenpox complications occur in less than 50 children per year. The risk of death from chickenpox in normal children is 0.0014 percent (Preblud, 1986). Children with a disease that compromises the immune system are more likely to develop complications from chickenpox. These children include cancer and leukemia patients undergoing chemotherapy and those with inborn immune deficiencies.

Adults who contract chickenpox generally have a more prolonged and serious illness. The complication rate is also higher in adults than in children. A severe form of encephalitis occurs more commonly in adults. This diffuse encephalitis is associated with a high mortality rate (5 to 35 percent). Women who contract chickenpox during the first 16 weeks of pregnancy may have children with congenital malformations. The estimated risk in one study of 150 women infected during pregnancy was less than 1 percent (Siegel *et al.*, 1966). Babies who are born within five days of their mother contracting chickenpox have a high risk of death. Severe illness often occurs in these babies during the first five to ten days after birth. The risk of death is estimated at 31 percent (Meyers, 1974).

Varicella Vaccine

A chickenpox vaccine was developed in 1973. As of this writing it is commonly used only in children with cancer and leukemia. Studies are continually being conducted to determine proper dosage, reactions, and effectiveness in normal children. Recent studies have evaluated the use of the vaccine in combination with the measles, mumps and rubella shot. It is relatively certain that the chickenpox vaccine will soon be added to those routinely administered to children. The MMRV (Measles, Mumps, Rubella, and Varicella) vaccine will replace MMR. The millions of dollars spent by drug manufacturers on varicella vaccine research will only be turned into profit if the vaccine is recommended for normal children. The drug companies will not patiently wait for a lifetime of study.

Vaccine Efficacy

The vaccine seems to be at least 90 percent effective in producing antibodies to the varicella-zoster virus (Arbeter, 1986). These antibodies persist at protective levels for several years. The persistence of immunity over longer periods has not been determined because the vaccine has not been tested in large enough trials for long enough periods of time. Vaccine tests have so far involved hundreds, rather than thousands, of children. The true test will come as soon as the vaccine is in common use.

We can attempt to predict the results of mass chickenpox vaccine usage from our experience with measles and mumps vaccines. Just as those diseases have become increasingly more prevalent in adults compared to children, with more likelihood of serious disease and resulting complications, so we are likely to see chickenpox become more common in adults. Persistence of vaccine effectiveness may decline over time. Unusual cases of varicella-zoster illness may also occur, as they do after measles and mumps vaccine. These possible effects are unknown, but they do concern vaccine researchers. Dr. Philip Brunell, in his introduction to a state-of-the-art report on varicella vaccine, describes the reluctance to use the vaccine in normal children because "chickenpox, which is relatively mild in childhood, might increase in frequency during adult life when it is much more severe" (Brunell, 1986). The experience with measles and mumps would seem to justify this cautionary note. Vaccine researcher Dr. Anne Gershon has stated this concern in even stronger terms:

One would not, however, want to vaccinate against varicella routinely in childhood if immunity wanes and thereby creates a population of varicella-susceptible adults. Long-term studies with a 3-10 year follow-up, but of only ≈ 100 vaccinees, suggest that antibody will be persistent. Practically, however, the only means to determine whether waning immunity will be a problem is to immunize a large number of healthy children and follow them for many years. Therefore, only post-licensure surveillance of immunized children can be utilized to determine if this will be a significant problem (Gershon, 1987).

After another massive experiment, the vaccine may prove to be a failure and then be withdrawn from routine use. Experimenting with the lives of thousands of people could be a colossal mistake.

Vaccine Reactions

Reactions to the vaccine in the very limited studies have been relatively mild. The most common reaction has been a generalized rash that resembles naturally acquired chickenpox. This eruption occurs in at least 5 to 10 percent of vaccinees (Arbeter, 1986). The eruption has been spread to susceptible contacts of vaccinees. In studies of vaccinated children with leukemia, 2 to 10 percent of siblings developed varicella vaccine virus eruptions (Gershon, 1984; Gershon, 1986). No serious vaccine reactions have been reported in the studies done so far.

Two possible long-term effects of the vaccine are feared by researchers, herpes zoster and cancer. Varicella-zoster virus can be stored in nerve cells after natural chickenpox infection and cause a recurrence of infection sometime later in the person's life. This subsequent infection is known as herpes zoster or shingles. It consists of a very painful skin eruption (the Danish term is "Hell's fire") which may persist for several weeks. Varicella vaccine has caused zoster in normal children (Plotkin, 1988). The rate of incidence is unknown, and it may or may not be greater than zoster which follows naturally acquired chickenpox. No one knows the possible effects of latent vaccine virus stored within the nervous system. Varicella-zoster virus may be a cause of cancer. This association has never been proven, though varicella-zoster-infected human cells have transformed mouse cells to cancerous cells in a laboratory setting (Yamanishi *et al.*, 1981). The possible long-term effects of this herpesvirus vaccine remain unknown.

Mass immunization of children will be a monumental experiment. Once again we are injecting children with a live virus which can cause encephalitis and has the ability to remain latent for an entire lifetime. Dr. Stanley Plotkin, an eminent researcher in the varicella-vaccine field, repeats an all-too-familiar ominous refrain in the march towards increasing vaccine usage. "I believe we will soon be ready to determine the effects of varicella vaccination in the general population of children" (Plotkin, 1988). This experiment is being conducted on your children.

TABLE 11

Varicella (Chickenpox) Summary

1. Chickenpox is a mild disease of childhood; complications of the disease are rare in normal children.

2. Adults almost always have more severe infection than children, and disease complications are more common.

3. Long-term efficacy of the vaccine is unknown. Widespread vaccine usage may shift the age distribution of chickenpox from children to adults.

4. Side effects of the vaccine and long-term effects are unknown. They could be more serious than measles and mumps vaccines because the chickenpox virus is associated with cancer and herpes zoster.

Recommendations

Varicella vaccine has questionable usefulness and introduces a persisting live virus into the body which has unknown long-term side effects. I do not recommend its use in normal children because of these uncertainties.

Acellular Pertussis

The public outcry over the tragic side effects of the currently used whole-cell pertussis vaccine has spurred a search for safer immunizations. Drug manufacturers are being pressured to develop a vaccine with less severe reactions. This occurred in Japan and to a lesser extent in the United States. In 1981 the Japanese switched from a whole-cell pertussis vaccine to a more complex acellular vaccine, primarily because of public pressure. Parents began refusing to give their children the whole-cell vaccine. The "improved" acellular vaccine was introduced to quell fears about the shots since the supposedly toxic components were removed. This vaccine seems to cause less of the mild-type reactions compared to the version currently used in the United States. In Japan the replacement of whole-cell with acellular vaccine resulted in a 60 percent reduction of "mild" side effects, particularly febrile seizures. But the rate of severe reactions did not differ significantly between the acellular and whole-cell vaccine (Noble *et al.*, 1987). The Japanese experience with acellular vaccine has included only children 24 months or older. There are no data that allow us to predict the rate of severe reactions for infants given the new vaccine (Cherry *et al.*, 1988).

A recent study in Sweden also revealed that the acellular vaccine also caused less of the mild-type side effects than the whole-cell vaccine. But severe systemic reactions did occur with the acellular vaccine. A total of 212 infants received the acellular vaccine. Two serious reactions occurred. These reactions are identical to those following the whole-cell vaccine. The case descriptions are quoted here at length.

Case 1. A girl who had received two doses of the acellular vaccine as primary immunization started to cry persistently 7 hours after the booster injection. The parents had never heard such a cry before. She cried for 1½ to 2 hours, and then went to bed and slept normally. The following morning she was found in bed pale, hypotonic, and unresponsive.

Case 2. A boy who had received three doses of the acellular vaccine as primary immunization became fretful, tired, and refused to eat 2 to 3 hours after the booster injection. The unusual behavior of the child continued, and he was hospitalized the following day. These symptoms recurred periodically during the 4 days of hospitalization. Clinical and laboratory examinations yielded no signs of infection or hypoglycemia. The boy recovered fully. Two EEGs [studies of brain waves] showed pathologic activity. The diagnosis was focal encephalitis of unknown origin (Blennow and Granstrom, 1989).

These limited studies of the acellular vaccine reveal that children immunized during infancy have serious vaccine reactions. In the Swedish study the rate of serious reactions was 1 in 100 vaccinated children. The limited scope of this study does not allow us to draw conclusions about frequency of severe reactions, but this rate is much *higher* than that reported for the current whole-cell vaccine.

The pertussis vaccine is dangerous in all forms developed thus far. The Japanese experience with use of acellular vaccine beginning at 2 years of age shows that reactions are significantly reduced if immunization is delayed, whether whole-cell vaccine or acellular vaccine is used. Infants will continue to be severely damaged by these pertussis vaccines, and the true extent of undetected, long-term disease will probably never be discovered.

TABLE 12

Acellular Pertussis Vaccine Summary

1. Severe reactions to the whole-cell pertussis vaccine have spurred worldwide efforts to produce a safer vaccine.

2. The acellular form of the pertussis vaccine seems to diminish mild-type reactions compared to the whole-cell vaccine.

3. Severe reactions to the acellular vaccine also occur.

Pneumococcal Vaccine

Streptococcus pneumonia (pneumococcus) is a bacterium associated with many cases of pneumonia, meningitis, bacteremia (systemic infection in the bloodstream), and ear infections. At least 10 to 25 percent of all pneumonias culture *S pneumonia* (Williams *et al.*, 1988) and approximately one-third of all ear infections in children are associated with *S pneumonia* growth (Bluestone and Klein, 1988). In addition, the estimated incidence of pneumococcal meningitis is 1 or 2 per 100,000 persons, and pneumococcal bacteremia (infection in the bloodstream) may occur as often as 160 per 100,000 for children under two years of age (MMWR, 1989h). The frequent encounters with pneumococcal disease have spurred a search for an effective vaccine. The bacterium has also become increasingly resistant to antibiotics, and this has further stimulated vaccine research.

Several pneumococcal vaccines are under investigation. In 1977 a pneumococcal vaccine was licensed which contained 14 types of *S pneumonia*. This was replaced by a vaccine of 23 types in 1983. These polysaccharide vaccines have met with limited success and new vaccine technology is under investigation. The polysaccharide has been bonded to a protein carrier to produce a conjugate vaccine that researchers hope will be more successful. Undoubtedly, this new vaccine will be included in the growing list of routine immunizations. Children will probably one day routinely receive the DTP-HIB-E-IPV-MMRV and PPP (Protein-Polysaccharide Pneumococcal) shot. This is not just a fantasy. Experts in vaccine research have stated, "It is conceivable that within a few years polysaccharide conjugate vaccines including four or more pneumococcal types, *H. influenzae* type b, and one or more meningococcal groups will be administered with diphtheria and tetanus toxoid and pertussis vaccine to children as young as two months of age" (Bluestone and Klein, 1988, p. 194).

The estimated effectiveness of the pneumococcal vaccine is 60 to 70 percent (MMWR, 1989h). However, four studies found little or no effect from the vaccine (Austrian, 1981; Simberkoff *et al.*, 1986; Forrester *et al.*, 1987). Most of the studies have been conducted in high-risk adult patients who are most susceptible to pneumonia. Studies of children reveal that the currently licensed polysacccharide vaccine is ineffective in children under 2 years of age.

Investigations of the pneumococcal vaccine for prevention of ear infections were begun in 1975. Results of three studies showed that vaccinated children had significantly fewer episodes of ear infections associated with the types of *S pneumonia* present in the vaccine. But children in the vaccine and control groups had the same number of ear infections. In other words, the vaccine did not prevent ear infections; it only altered the types of microbes present in the ear (Karma *et al.*, 1980; Makela, *et al.*, 1980, 1981; Sloyer *et al.*, 1981; Teele *et al.*, 1981). The vaccine currently is not recommended for prevention of ear infections.

The only children who now routinely receive the pneumococcal vaccine are those at increased risk of serious pneumococcal infections. This group includes those children with certain chronic diseases that impair the immune system, and those who have had their spleen removed (MMWR, 1989h).

The vaccine has been associated with few side effects. Approximately 50 percent of vaccinees (30 to 40 percent in children) develop swelling and pain at the injection site. Fever, muscle pain, and severe swelling occur in less than one percent of those vaccinated. High fevers (over 102°) and severe allergic reactions have been reported (Committee on Infectious Diseases, 1985).

TABLE 13
Pneumococcal Vaccine Summary

1. *Streptococcus pneumonia* is associated with a large percentage of ear infections, meningitis, pneumonia, and bacteremia in children.

2. The currently licensed vaccine is 60 to 70 percent effective in preventing serious disease.

3. Studies do not show any appreciable effect on reduction of ear infections in children.

4. Vaccine is currently recommended for children with chronic diseases and not for normal children.

Recommendations

Soon the pneumococcal vaccine will be available for all children. It will be deemed safe and effective in preventing pneumonia, meningitis, and ear infections. It will probably be combined with other vaccines as part of the recommended immunization schedule. This will occur regardless of its low rate of effectiveness. Hib vaccine is already recommended for all children despite its very poor protective capacity.

The long-term effects of the pneumococcal vaccine are unknown. They will only be discovered if severe reactions occur soon after injection. Otherwise the effects of this vaccine will be inextricably combined with those of other routine immunizations of childhood and we will never know whether there are deleterious effects or not. The same possibilities exist for this vaccine as with the other bacteria and viruses that have neurotoxic effects (pertussis, *Hemophilus*, measles). They all could cause encephalitis and contribute to the brain injury syndrome postulated by Coulter. I cannot recommend this vaccine for normal children.

Conclusion

Most parents take the issue of immunizations for granted. The pediatrician says their children need them, and so they do it. Parents may have misgivings and may not like the idea, but they often have no support for these feelings. The pediatrician is a powerful influence on parents, and most pediatricians are committed to the campaign for universal immunization. But questions about immunization are far from completely answered. Questions of efficacy, risks, and long-term effects remain troubling issues for vaccine researchers.

Some parents are philosophically opposed to the concept of vaccinating their children. They are more horrified by the idea of injecting poisonous substances into their child than they are concerned about the remote future possibility of the diseases. For these parents the vaccines represent a dangerous form of Russian roulette they are unwilling to play.

Other parents may be anxious about the effects of vaccines on their child, but they are concerned that if enough people avoid the shots then the diseases will begin to reappear. The vaccines may have bad side effects, but if I avoid them for my child then the vaccine campaign will not work for the general population. This is a sacrificial philosophy. Risk the side effects in my child for the good of the whole society. The stakes of this game may be exceedingly high if the vaccines are capable of causing a covert encephalitis syndrome. If that is true, then we are trading one disease for another. This sacrifice is hardly worth the cost.

I assume that most parents who have read this book are concerned about the side effects of vaccines. Most parents are also anxious about some of the diseases discussed here. In fact, for parents the impetus to give vaccines is primarily based on anxiety. What if one of these diseases should happen to my unvaccinated child? The potential guilt factor is tremendous. Never mind that some of the vaccines have very questionable efficacy themselves. If parents do vaccinate, then at least they eliminate the guilt if a child contracts a disease. So one of the main tasks for parents to accomplish when they choose not to vaccinate is overcoming anxiety and guilt. But imagine the guilt and self-reproach if your child is severely damaged by a vaccine.

Anxiety about disease is a serious issue for parents. Tetanus is the best example. Parents who choose not to get tetanus shots for their children often think about cuts and puncture wounds. When little Josh climbs up the slide, they wonder about tetanus bacteria in the fertilized soil of the playground. This is enough to distract a parent from enjoying playtime.

Exposure to other children may cause anxiety for parents of unvaccinated children for two reasons. First, you may worry that your child could be exposed to children who bring diseases from other countries. Parents especially worry about polio and whooping cough. Parents should keep in mind the figures cited in the polio section of this book. No cases of polio have occurred in the United States since 1979. This includes immigrants, aliens, and visitors from other countries. Your child cannot contract a disease unless he or she is exposed to one. Other diseases, such as measles and mumps, do exist in the United States, but exposure to them may be beneficial to your child, providing lifelong immunity. The pertussis vaccine, in my opinion, has too many associated side effects to risk its use in your child, regardless of exposure to the disease.

The second anxiety about your unvaccinated child's exposure to others concerns polio. Children who are immunized early in life with the oral, live vaccine may shed the virus in their stools. Exposure of your child to recently vaccinated children is a potential hazard. Parents should keep in mind that more than 95 percent of cases of illness caused by the polio virus manifest as a cold. Nonetheless, the risk is there. Parents should be vocal about their concerns. Ask whether playmates and other children in daycare have recently received the oral polio vaccine. It is appropriate for other parents to be concerned that their vaccinated children could spread the disease to others. They should be educated about this possibility, and assume responsibility for limiting the likelihood of their child spreading the virus to unvaccinated children. In the future the likelihood of this exposure will diminish because babies will be immunized with the killed (E-IPV) polio vaccine, which does not cause polio in recipients or contacts.

The only way for parents of unvaccinated children to feel secure is to remember the reasons for their decision in the first place. Parents often need booster doses of vaccine education. They should keep in mind three points of information:

(1) Vaccines have immediate, sometimes drastic, side effects.

(2) Vaccines have unknown long-term side effects which may include post-encephalitis brain damage.

(3) Vaccine efficacy may decrease over time, making children susceptible to the viral diseases as adults when the diseases are more serious.

Parents of unvaccinated children should expect that they will be continually harassed and reproached about their child's "immunization status." Kindred friends may help to offer support, but the concerns of family members themselves can be almost overwhelming. Grandparents are notorious worriers. Their well-intentioned concern should be politely ignored. At best, parents can offer books like this one or those in the

Resources section to troubled family members. If two spouses disagree about vaccination and reach an impasse, then I recommend that the spouse opposed to the vaccines firmly hold her ground. There is no more tenacious an animal than a mother protecting her child from harm. If you are convinced that vaccines present a significant threat to your child's health, then do not allow them. No one can inject vaccines without your consent. Withhold your consent if you have serious doubts about their safety and advisability.

Schools will provide a continual source of difficulty to parents of unvaccinated children. Again, parents should simply hold firm in their resolve. Seek out a medical provider who is willing to sign a medical release. Any doctor who suspects that vaccines may have long-term damaging effects should be willing to sign a letter stating that vaccines are medically contraindicated. School district personnel in states that offer a religious or philosophical exemption may need to be educated about this option. Provide them with information about your state's laws governing immunization exemptions. You will be paving the way for another parent in your position. Colleges and universities also require immunizations, and the same rules apply as for other schools. No child should be immunized against a parent's better judgment. Legal protection is available against forced vaccination. If necessary, seek the services of a knowledgeable attorney (see Resources).

The final frontier in communicating your decision about immunizations is the pediatrician or family physician. These doctors care for your child, medically and emotionally. They should be a source of support for you and your child. They may disagree with your decision and voice their concerns, but they should respect your opinions and judgments. Talk with them about your concerns, show them that you are knowledgeable about vaccine side effects and disease incidence. Share this book with them. Do your part in communicating. They will benefit from your insights. If you meet with hostility or terminal resistance, then you may want to seek another medical provider who is more receptive and understanding. I know pediatricians who are. I also know pediatricians who post notes in their offices stating, "If you don't immunize, don't bring your child to me for care." Do not give up and do not be intimidated. Your physician is working for you as part of a team that cares for your child. You are the manager of that team.

If you have made an educated and informed decision not to vaccinate your child, then you can be proud of your choice. Remember that doubts often plague parents who choose to vaccinate. They wonder if they did the right thing. Should they continue with boosters once they have started? All those other shots might be wasted. If you have doubts at any point, you can stop giving the vaccines. Remember that vaccines often cause severe reactions only after the third or fourth shot. The doubts of parents with unvaccinated children are even stronger. Am I risking my child's life when he is exposed to strangers or children from "other cultures" playing in the park? Parents can never be sure they are doing the right thing. But if your doubts about the safety of the vaccine campaign are strong enough, then it makes sense to allow your child's body to fight off diseases and develop a strong immune system capable of handling infectious disease on its own. This may be one of the greatest gifts you give to your child.

Immunization Schedule

The following schedules for immunization have been included so that parents will know what to expect from health providers who recommend the vaccines. Again, it is important to remember that immunizations can be delayed and given at any time parents prefer. Parents can choose to give some vaccines and not others. If you decide to give the vaccines, the tetanus, diphtheria, pertussis, or polio vaccines should be given as a series, in order to achieve recommended antibody levels.

DTP = Diphtheria and Tetanus Toxoids and Pertussis Vaccine

HbCV = Hemophilus influenzae b polysaccharide antigen conjugated to a protein carrier

MMR = Measles, Mumps, and Rubella Virus Vaccine Live

OPV = Poliovirus Vaccine Live Oral, Trivalent

Td = Tetanus and Diphtheria Toxoids

TABLE 14
Immunization Schedule for Infants

2 mos.	DTP #1, OPV #1
4 mos.	DTP #2, OPV #2
6 mos.	DTP #3
15 mos.	MMR, DTP #4, OPV #3
18 mos.	HbCV
4-6 yrs.	DTP #5, OPV #4
14-16 yrs.	Td

TABLE 15
Immunization Schedule for Children up to 7 Years Old

First visit	DTP #1, OPV #1
	MMR (if ≥15 mos)
	HbCV (if ≥18 mos)
2 mos later	DTP #2, OPV #2
4 mos later	DTP #3
6-12 mos after DPT #3	DTP #4, OPV #3
Preschool (4-6 yrs)	DTP #5, OPV #4
14-16 yrs	Td

TABLE 16
Immunization Schedule for Children over 7 Years Old

First visit	Td #1, OPV #1, MMR
2 mos later	Td #2, OPV #2
6-12 mos after Td #2	Td #3, OPV #3
10 yrs after Td #3	Td

Resources

Organizations
Dissatisfied Parents Together (DPT)
An organization of concerned lay people and professionals that promotes information about vaccines and assists parents in their legal battles to obtain compensation for vaccine injury, avoid immunization in situations where legal pressures are applied, and promote legislation relating to safe immunizations and free choice. Members receive a regular newsletter.

128 Branch Road
Vienna, VA 22180
(703) 938-DPT3

National Center for Homeopathy
Information resource center for homeopathic medicine. They publish a national directory of homeopathic practitioners.

1500 Massachusetts Ave N.W., Suite 42
Washington, D.C. 20005
(202) 223-6182

Homeopathic Educational Services
A distributor and mail-order supplier of homeopathic books, audiotapes and summaries of homeopathic research. Send for catalog.

2124 Kittredge St.
Berkeley, CA 94704
(415) 653-9270

Reprints of articles

Richard Moskowitz, MD *The Case Against Immunizations*
A fascinating theoretical investigation of vaccine side-effects with emphasis on their possible role in immune system dysfunction. Fairly technical.

National Center for Homeopathy
1500 Massachusetts Ave N.W., Suite 42
Washington, D.C. 20005
(202) 223-6182

Immunizations
A collection of articles from *Mothering* reprinted in booklet form. These give a wide-ranging view, including articles by physicians and parents about many areas of concern to parents who must make the immunization decision.

Mothering Magazine
PO Box 8410
Santa Fe, NM 87504
(505) 984-8116

Immunization articles by Robert Mendelsohn, MD
A collection of articles by the late pediatrician, Dr. Mendelsohn, one of the most outspoken critics of vaccines. He was unequivocally opposed to immunizations and a reassuring voice to parents who have opted to avoid the vaccines.

The Doctor's People
1578 Sherman Ave, Suite 318
Evanston, IL 60201

Books

Coulter, H.L. *The Assault on the American Child: Vaccination, Sociopathy, and Criminality*, North Atlantic Books, Berkeley, California, 1990.
Describes childhood immunizations as a possible cause of encephalitis characterized by learning problems, developmental delays, behavior disorders, and autism.

Coulter, H.L. & Fisher, B.L. *DPT: A Shot in the Dark*, Harcourt, Brace, Jovanovich Publishers, Orlando, Florida, 1985.
Documentation of the devastating effects of the pertussis vaccine, including vivid case examples and an exposé of the campaign for mandatory immunization of children regardless of the risks.

Cummings, S., Ullman, D. *Everybody's Guide to Homeopathic Medicines*, Jeremy P Tarcher, Inc., Los Angeles, 1984.
An introduction to homeopathic principles and the use of homeopathic medicines to treat the common acute illnesses of children and adults.

James, W. *Immunization: The Reality Behind the Myth*, Bergin & Garvey Publishers, Granberry, Massachusetts, 1988.
A description of the problems with immunization statistics and a proposal for parents to build a strong immune system in their children without using vaccines.

Mendelsohn, R. *How to Raise a Healthy Child . . . In Spite of Your Doctor*, Contemporary Books, Chicago, 1984.
A practical and common-sense guide advising parents to avoid overtreatment, immunizations, and other hazards encountered in the pediatrician's office.

References

AAP News; Vaccine brochures: AAP proposes changes. June 1989, p 2.

Albrecht, P., Ennis, F.A., Saltzman, E.J., Krugman, S. Persistence of maternal antibody in infants beyond 12 months: mechanisms of measles vaccine failure. *Journal of Pediatrics* 1977; 91:715-718.

Alderslade, R., Bellman, M.H., Rawson, N.S., et al., The National Childhood Encephalopathy Study, in *Whooping Cough: Reports from the Committee on Safety of Medicines and the Joint Committee on Vaccination and Immunisation*. London, Department of Health and Social Security, Her Majesty's Stationery Office, 1981, pp 79-154.

American Institute of Homeopathy. *Special Report of the Homeopathic Yellow Fever Commission Ordered by the AIH for Presentation to Congress*. Philadelphia and New York; Boericke and Tafel, 1880.

Arbeter, A.M., Starr, S.E., Plotkin, S.A. Varicella vaccine studies in healthy children and adults. *Pediatrics* 1986; 78(suppl):748-756.

Austrian, R. *Review of Infectious Disease* 1981; 3(suppl):S1-S17.

Baraff, L.J., Ablon, W.J., Weiss, R.C. Possible temporal association between diphtheria-tetanus toxoid-pertussis vaccination and sudden infant death syndrome. *Pediatric Infectious Disease Journal* 1983; 2:7-11.

Bart, K.J., Orenstein, W.A., Preblud, S.R., Hinman, A.R. Universal immunization to interrupt rubella. *Review of Infectious Disease* 1985; 7(suppl 1):S177-184.

Berkowitz, C.D., Ward, J.I., Meier, K., et al. Persistence of antibody (AB) to Haemophilus influenzae type b (Hib) and response to PRP amd PRP-D booster immunization in children initially immunized with either vaccine at 15 to 24 months (Abstract no. 889). *Pediatric Research* 1987; 21:321A.

Blennow, M., and Granstrom, M. Adverse reactions and serologic response to a booster dose of acellular pertussis vaccine in children immunized with acellular or whole-cell vaccine as infants. *Pediatrics* 1989; 84:62-67.

Bluestone, C.D., and Klein, J.O. *Otitis Media in Infants and Children*. W.B. Saunders Company, Philadelphia, 1988.

Bradford, T.L. *The Logic of Figures or Comparative Results of Homeopathic and Other Treatments*. Boericke and Tafel, Philadelphia, 1900.

Broome, C.V., Epidemiology of Haemophilus influenzae type b infections in the United States. *Pediatric Infectious Disease Journal* 1987; 6:779-782.

Brunell, P.A. Varicella vaccine - Where are we? *Pediatrics* 1986; 78(suppl):721-722.

Castro, D., and Nogueira, G.G. Use of the nosode Meningococcinum as a preventive against meningitis. *Journal of the American Institute of Homeopathy* 1975; 68:211-219.

Chandra, R.K. Immunological aspects of human milk. *Nutrition Review* 1978; 36:265.

Cherry, J.D., Feigin, R.D., Lobes, L.A., Shackelford, P.G. Atypical measles in children previously immunized with attenuated measles virus vaccines. *Pediatrics* 1972; 50:712.

Cherry, J.D., Brunell, P.A., Golden, G.S., Karzon, D.T. Report of the task force on pertussis and pertussis immunization—1988. *Pediatrics* 1988; 81 (suppl):939-984.

Church, J.A, and Richards, W. Recurrent abscess formation following DTP immunizations: association with hypersensitivity to tetanus toxoid. *Pediatrics* 1985; 75:899-900.

Cochi, S.L., Preblud, S.R., Orenstein, W.A. Perspectives on the relative resurgence of mumps in the United States. *American Journal of Diseases of Children* 1988; 142:499-507.

Cody, C.L., Baraff, L.J., Cherry, J.D., et al. Nature and rates of adverse reactions associated with DTP and DT immunizations in infants and children. *Pediatrics* 1981; 68:650-660.

Committee on Infectious Diseases, American Academy of Pediatrics. Measles: Reassessment of the current immunization policy. *Pediatrics* 1989; 84:1110-1113.

Committee on Infectious Diseases, American Academy of Pediatrics. Recommendations for using pneumococcal vaccine in children. *Pediatrics* 1985; 75:1153-1158.

Coulter, H.L. *The Assault on the American Child: Vaccination, Sociopathy, and Criminality*, North Atlantic Books, Berkeley, California, 1990.

Coulter, H.L., and Fisher, B.L. *DPT: A Shot in the Dark*, Harcourt, Brace, Jovanovich Publishers, Orlando, Florida, 1985.

Crowder, M., Higgins, H.L., Frost, J.J. Rubella susceptibility in young women of rural east Texas: 1980 and 1985. *Texas Medicine* 1987; 83:43-47.

Dodge, P.R., Davis, H., Feigin, R.D., et al. Prospective evaluation of hearing impairment as a sequelae of acute bacterial meningitis. *New England Journal of Medicine* 1984; 311:869-874.

Edsall, G. Specific prophylaxis of tetanus. *Journal of the American Medical Association* 1959; 171:417-427.

Eisfelder, H.W. Poliomyelitis immunization—a final report. *Journal of the American Institute of Homeopathy* 1961; 54:166-167.

English, J.M. (a) Pertussin 30—preventive for whooping cough? A pilot study. *British Homeopathic Journal* 1987; 76:61-65.

English, J.M. (b) Symptoms and treatment of whooping cough, 1980-1982. *British Homeopathic Journal* 1987; 76:66-68.

Faculty review of Asian influenza. *Homeopathy* 1958; 8:115-124.

Eskola, J., Peltola, H., Takala, A.K., et al. Efficacy of Haemophilus influenzae type b polysaccharide-diphtheria toxoid conjugate vaccine in infancy. *New England Journal of Medicine* 1987; 317:717-722.

Feldman, H.M., and Michaels, R.H. Academic achievement in children ten to 12 years after *Haemophilus influenzae* meningitis. *Pediatrics* 1988; 81:339-344.

Fenichel, G.M. Neurological complications of immunization. *Annals of Neurology* 1982; 12:119-128.

Forrester, H.L., Jahnigen, D.W., LaForce, F.M. Inefficacy of pneumococcal vaccine in a high-risk population. *American Journal of Medicine* 1987; 83:425-430.

Fulginiti, V.A. Controversies in current immunization policies and practices. *Current Problems in Pediatrics* 1976; 6:6-16.

Gershon, A.A., Steinberg, S., Galasso, G., *et al.* Live attenuated varicella vaccine in children with leukemia in remission. *Biken Journal* 1984; 27:77.

Gershon, A.A., Steinberg, S.P., Gelb, L. Live attenuated varicella vaccine use in immunocompromised children and adults. *Pediatrics* 1986; 78(suppl):757-762.

Gershon, A.A. Live attenuated varicella vaccine. *Annual Review of Medicine* 1987; 38:41-50.

Gilmartin, R.C., Jabbour, J.T., Duenas, D.A. Rubella vaccine myeloradiculoneuritis. *Journal of Pediatrics* 1972; 80:406-412.

Goldman, A.S., et al. Immunologic factors in human milk during the first year of lactation. *Journal of Pediatrics* 1982; 100:563.

Guess, H.A., Broughton, D.D., Melton, L.J., Kurland, L.T. Population-based studies of varicella complications. *Pediatrics* 1986; 78(suppl):723-727.

Gunderson, J.R. Guillain-Barré syndrome: Occurrence following combined mumps-rubella vaccine. *American Journal of Diseases of Childhood* 1973; 125:834-835.

Gustafson, T.L., Lievens, A.W., Brunell, P.A., et al. Measles outbreak in a fully immunized secondary-school population. *New England Journal of Medicine* 1987; 316:771-774.

Harrison, L.H., Broome, C.V., Hightower, M.S. *Haemophilus influenzae* type b polysaccharide vaccine: an efficacy study. *Pediatrics* 1989; 84:255-261.

Intensive Immunization Programs. *Hearings before the Committee on Interstate and Foreign Commerce, House of Representatives, 87th Congress, 2nd Session on H.R. 10541*. US Government Printing Office, Washington, DC, 1962.

Hough, J.C., et al. Rubella seroconversion following immunization in a rural practice. *Journal of Family Practice* 1979; 9:587-589.

Hull, H.F., Montes, J.M., Hays, P.C., Lucero, R.L. Risk factors for measles vaccine failure among immunized students. *Pediatrics* 1985; 76:518-523.

Institute of Medicine. An Evaluation of Poliomyelitis Vaccine Policy Options. National Academy of Sciences, Washington,

DC, 1988. IOM publication 88-04.

JAMA (Journal of the American Medical Association) 1959; 170:142-143, 2246-2247.

James, W. *Immunization: The Reality Behind the Myth*, Bergin & Garvey Publishers, Granberry, Massachusetts, 1988.

Johnson, D.M. Fatal tetanus after prophylaxis with human tetanus immune globulin. *Journal of the American Medical Association* 1969; 207:1519.

Kaplan, S.L., and Fishman, M.A. Update on bacterial meningitis. *Journal of Child Neurology* 1988; 3:82-93.

Karma, P., Luotonen, J., Timonen, M., *et al.* Efficacy of pneumococcal vaccination against recurrent otitis media. Preliminary results of a field trial in Finland. *Annals of Otology, Rhinology, and Laryngology* 1980; 89:357-362.

Kilroy, A.W. Two syndromes following rubella immunization. *Journal of the American Medical Association* 1970; 214:2287-2292.

Lambert, H. Epidemiology of a small pertussis outbreak in Kent County, Michigan. *Public Health Reports* 1965; 80:365-369.

Makela, P.H., Sibakov, M., Herva, E., Henricksen, J. Pneumococcal vaccine and otitis media. *Lancet* 1980; 2:547-551.

Makela, P.H., Leinonen, M., Tukander, J., Karma, P. A study of the pneumococcal vaccine in prevention of clinically acute attacks of recurrent otitis media. *Review of Infectious Disease* 1981; 3:S124-S130.

Marcuse, E.K. Why wait for DTP-E-IPV? *American Journal of Diseases of Children* 1989; 143:1006-1007.

Markowitz, L.E., Preblud, S.R., Orenstein, W.A., *et al.* Patterns of transmission in measles outbreaks in the United States, 1985-1986. *New England Journal of Medicine* 1989; 320:75-81.

Marshall, G.S., Wright, P.F., Fenichel, G.M., Karzon, D.T. Diffuse retinopathy following measles, mumps, and rubella vaccination. *Pediatrics* 1985; 76:989-991.

McComb, J.A., and Dwyer, R.C. Passive-active immunization with tetanus immune globulin (human). *New England Journal of Medicine* 1963; 268:857-862.

McComb, J.A., and Levine, L. Adult immunization: dosage reduction as a solution to increasing reactions to tetanus toxoid. *New England Journal of Medicine* 1961; 265:1152-1153.

Mendelsohn, R. The truth about immunizations. *The People's Doctor* April 1978, p. 1.

Meyers, J.D. Congenital varicella in term infants: Risk reconsidered. *Journal of Infectious Disease* 1974; 129:215-217.

Milstien, J.B., Gross, T.P., Kuritsky, J.N. Adverse reactions reported following receipt of Haemophilus influenzae type b vaccine: an analysis after 1 year of marketing. *Pediatrics* 1987; 80:270-274.

MMWR (Morbidity and Mortality Weekly Report), Tetanus— United States, 1982-1985. 1985; 34: 602, 607-611.

MMWR (Morbidity and Mortality Weekly Report), International notes: Imported paralytic poliomyelitis—United States, 1986. 1986; 35:671-674.

MMWR (Morbidity and Mortality Weekly Report), Tetanus— United States, 1986-1986. 1987; 36:477-481.

MMWR (Morbidity and Mortality Weekly Report), Prevention of Haemophilus influenzae type b disease. 1988; 37:13-16.

MMWR (Morbidity and Mortality Weekly Report), Measles— Quebec. 1989(a); 38:329-330.

MMWR (Morbidity and Mortality Weekly Report), ACIP: General recommendation on immunization. 1989(b); 38:205-227.

MMWR (Morbidity and Mortality Weekly Report), Measles—
Los Angeles County, California, 1988. 1989(c); 38:49-57.

MMWR (Morbidity and Mortality Weekly Report), ACIP:
Measles prevention: supplementary statement. 1989(d); 38:11-
14.

MMWR (Morbidity and Mortality Weekly Report), Measles—
United States, 1988. 1989(i); 38:601-605.

MMWR (Morbidity and Mortality Weekly Report), Mumps—
United States, 1985-1988. 1989(e); 38:101-105.

MMWR (Morbidity and Mortality Weekly Report), Rubella and
congenital rubella syndrome—United States, 1985-1988.
1989(f) 38:173-178.

MMWR (Morbidity and Mortality Weekly Report), Mumps prevention. 1989(g) 38:388-400.

MMWR (Morbidity and Mortality Weekly Report), Pneumococcal polysaccharide vaccine. 1989(h); 38:64-76.

Mortimer, E.A. Immunization against infectious disease.
Science 1978; 200:902.

Moskowitz, R. The case against immunizations. *Journal of the
American Institute of Homeopathy* 1983; 76:7-25.

Moskowitz, R. Immunizations: the other side. *Mothering*
1984; 31:32-38.

Nightingale, E.O. Recommendations for a national policy on
poliomyelitis vaccination. *New England Journal of Medicine*
1977; 297:249-253

Noble, G.R., Bernier, R.H., Esber, E.C., *et al*. Acellular and
whole-cell pertussis vaccines in Japan: Report of a visit by US
scientists. *Journal of the American Medical Association* 1987;
257:1351-1356.

Osterholm, M.T., *et al*. Lack of efficacy of Haemophilus b

References   105

polysaccharide vaccine in Minnesota. *Journal of the American Medical Association* 1988; 260:1423-1428.

Pate, J.E. *The School Performance of Post Haemophilus influenzae Meningitic Children: Dallas. Final Report.* Education Resources Information Center, E.D. 067801, U.S. Office of Education, July 1, 1972.

Philip, R.N., Reinhard, K.R., Lackman, D.B. Observations on a mumps epidemic in a "virgin" population. *American Journal of Hygiene* 1959; 69:91-111.

Plotkin, S. Hell's fire and varicella-vaccine safety. *New England Journal of Medicine* 1988; 318:573-575.

Pollock, T.M., and Morris, J. A 7-year survey of disorders attributed to vaccination in Northwest Thames Region. *Lancet* 1983; 1:753-757.

Preblud, S.R. Varicella: complications and costs. *Pediatrics* 1986; 78(suppl):728-735.

Relihan, M. Reactions to tetanus toxoid. *Journal of the American Medical Association* 1969; 62:430-434.

St. Geme, J.W., George, B.L., Bush, B.M. Exaggerated natural measles following attenuated virus immunization. *Pediatrics* 1976; 57:148-150.

Schoenbaum, S.C., Biano, S., Mack, T. Epidemiology of congenital rubella syndrome: The role of maternal parity. *Journal of the American Medical Association* 1975; 233:151-155.

Sell, S.H. Haemophilus influenzae type b meningitis: manifestations and long-term sequelae. *Pediatric Infectious Disease Journal* 1987; 6:775-778.

Sell, S.H., Webb, W.W., Pate, J.E., *et al.* Psychological sequelae to bacterial meningitis: Two controlled studies. *Pediatrics* 1972; 49:212-217.

Shasby, D.M., Shope, T.C., Downs, H., Herrmann, K.L.,

Polkowski, J. Epidemic measles in a highly vaccinated population. *New England Journal of Medicine* 1977; 296:585-589.

Sieber, O.F., Fulginiti, V.A. Is adult immunization more appropriate than immunization of infants? *Pediatrics* 1977; 60:562-563.

Simberkoff, M.S., Cross, A.P., Al-Ibrahim, M., *et al.* Efficacy of pneumococcal vaccine in high-risk patients: results of a Veterans Administration cooperative study. *New England Journal of Medicine* 1986; 315:1316-1327.

Siegel, M., Fuerst, H.T., Peress, N.S. Comparative fetal mortality in maternal virus diseases: A prospective study on rubella, measles, mumps, chickenpox, and hepatitis. *New England Journal of Medicine* 1966; 274:768-771.

Skudder, P.A., and McCarroll, J.R. Current status of tetanus control: Importance of human tetanus-immune globulin. *Journal of the American Medical Association* 1964; 188:625-627.

Sloyer, J.L., Ploussard, J.H., Howie, V.M. Efficacy of pneumococcal polysaccharide vaccine in preventing acute otitis media in infants in Huntsville, Alabama. *Review of Infectious Disease* 1981; 3:S119-S123.

Teele, D.W., Pelton, S.I., Klein, J.O. Bacteriology of acute otitis media unresponsive to initial antimicrobial therapy. *Journal of Pediatrics* 1981; 98:537-539.

Tejani, A., Dobias, B., Sambursky, J. Long-term prognosis after H. influenzae meningitis: Prospective evaluation. *Developmental Medicine and Childhood Neurology* 1982; 24:338-343.

Torch, W. Diphtheria-pertussis-tetanus (DTP) immunization: A potential cause of the sudden infant death syndrome (SIDS). *Neurology* 1982; 32:A169.

Waler, A.M., Jick, H., Perera, D.R., *et al.* Diphtheria-tetanus-pertussis immunization and sudden infant death syndrome. *American Journal of Public Health* 1987; 77:945-951.

Ward, J. Newer Haemophilus influenzae type b vaccines and passive prophylaxis. *Pediatric Infectious Disease Journal* 1987; 6:799-803.

Weiner, L.B., Corwin, R.M., Nieburg, P.I., Feldman, H.A. A Measles outbreak among adolescents. *Journal of Pediatrics* 1977; 90:17-20.

White, F. Measles vaccine associated encephalitis in Canada. *Lancet* 1983; 2:683-684.

White, W.G., Barnes, G.M., Barker, E., *et al.* Reactions to tetanus toxoid. *Journal of Hygiene* 1983; 71:283-297.

Williams, W.W., Hickson, M.A., Kane, M.A., *et al.* Immunization policies and vaccine coverage among adults: the risk for missed opportunities. *Annals of Internal Medicine* 1988; 108:616-625.

Pertussis, susceptibility factors, 43-44
Pertussis whole cell vaccine, 80-81
Pharmaceutical manufacturers, 18, 48
Philosophical belief exemptions, 20, 87, 90
Placebo control group, 15, 45
Polio, wild, 38, 41
Pneumococcal bacteremia, 83
Pneumococcal disease, see Pneumonia
Pneumococcal meningitis, 68, 83
Pneumonia, 44, 53, 67-68, 73, 83-85, 99-100
Polio, 2-4, 16-19, 37-42, 73, 88-89, 92, 100- 101
Polio epidemics, 3, 37
Polio statistics, 16, 38-40, 42
Polio underdeveloped countries, 37
Polio vaccine, x
Poliovirus Vaccine Live Oral, Trivalent, 92
Polysaccharide vaccine, meningitis, 69
Polysaccharide vaccines, pneumonia, 83-84
Poor living conditions, 51
Poor self-control, 24
Positive reinforcement, 25
Postmeningitic children, 68
Postpubertal populations, 64
Post-licensure surveillance, 77
Post-vaccinal encephalitis, 46
Pregnancy, 62-66, 75
Prepared baby foods, 23
Private schools, 21
Processed foods, 23
Profit, 4, 72, 76
Proponents of vaccines, 10, 16, 18, 39
Protein carrier, 67, 83-84
Psychological sequelae to bacterial meningitis, 105
Public health authorities, 15, 55
Public health goal, 54
Public pressure, 80

Rashes, 62, 66, 70, 77
Reading problems, 68
Reduction of stress, 24
Refined and processed foods, 22-23
Relaxation, 24
Religious beliefs, 20
Religious or philosophical exemptions, 20-21, 90
Reporting practices by physicians, 39
Reprints of articles, 95
Research, 72, 83
Residual paralysis, 40
Resistance, 13, 22, 69
Resistance to infection, 13, 22, 24, 69

Resources Organizations, 94
Respiratory infection, 8, 30, 44
Respiratory paralysis, 38
Rest, 24
Retardation, 4, 8, 43, 47, 62
Retina, 56
Reye syndrome, 75
Rheumatoid arthritis, 65
Rotation diet, 23
Rubella, 52, 56, 62-66, 75-76, 92-99, 101-106
Runny nose, 74
Rural practice, 101
Russia, 11
Russian roulette, 87

Sabin vaccine, see Polio
Sacrificial philosophy, 87
Salivary gland, 59
Salk, see Polio
Sanitation, 15, 35
Sanitation practices, 24
Scarlet fever, 24
Schedules for immunization, 92-93
Scotland, 47
Screaming, 10
Second six months of life, 23
Secondary infections, 74
Sedatives, 31
Seizures, 4, 45, 56, 60, 67
Self-confidence, 25
Self-limited disease, 53
Self-reproach, 88
Sensory nerve deficits, 56, 65
Sequelae, 10; pertussis, 46; measles 56; meningitis 70; acute bacterial meningitis, 99
Serologic testing, 31, 51, 54, 63-64, 98, 105
Serum sickness, 70
Shingles, 77
Side effects see Vaccine reactions
SIDS, 45, 48, 97, 106
Skin, 30, 74, 77
Sleep, 24, 46
Smallpox, 3, 7, 24
Soft neurodevelopmental symptoms, 47
Sore throat, 38
South America, 11
Spasms, 30
Spinal paralytic poliomyelitis, see Polio
Spleen, 84
State Health Departments, 20-21
Statistics acellular pertussis, 80; bias and distortions, 15-16, 39-40; diptheria, 50-51; homeopathy, 12; measles, 54-55; meningitis, (Hib), 65, 68-69;

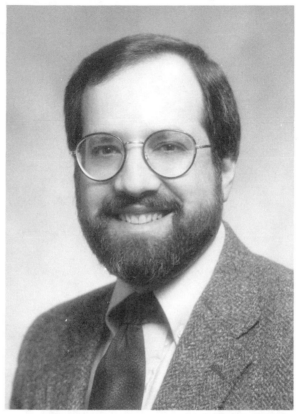

photo by Theodore H. Mock

Dr. Neustaedter practices homeopathic medicine in Palo Alto, California, specializing in child health care. A well-recognized author, his works include an authoritative text of *Homeopathic Pediatrics* and many articles in the homeopathic medical journals. Dr. Neustaedter was past director of the homeopathic medicine department at Pacific College of Naturopathic Medicine and lectures at the Hahnemann College of Homeopathy. He is a licensed acupuncturist and received his Doctorate in Oriental Medicine in Hong Kong. His practice integrates homeopathy, acupuncture, and modern diagnostic medicine.